Calm Energy

HOW PEOPLE REGULATE MOOD

Calm Energy

WITH FOOD AND EXERCISE

Robert E. Thayer, Ph.D.

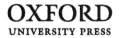

OXFORD
UNIVERSITY PRESS

OXFORD
UNIVERSITY PRESS

Oxford   New York
Auckland   Bangkok   Buenos Aires   Cape Town
Chennai   Dar es Salaam   Delhi   Hong Kong   Istanbul   Karachi
Kolkata   Kuala Lumpur   Madrid   Melbourne   Mexico City   Mumbai   Nairobi
São Paulo   Shanghai   Taipei   Tokyo   Toronto

First published by Oxford University Press, Inc., 2001
First issued as an Oxford University Press paperback, 2003
198 Madison Avenue, New York, New York 10016

www.oup.com

Oxford is a registered trademark of Oxford University Press

Library of Congress Cataloging-in-Publication Data
Thayer, Robert E.
Calm energy : how people regulate mood with food and exercise / Robert E. Thayer.
p. cm.
Includes bibliographical references and index.
ISBN-13 978-0-19-516339-1
1. Mental health—nutritional aspects.
2. Mood (Psychology).
3. Nutrition—Psychological aspects.
4. Exercise—Psychological aspects.
I. Title.

RC454.4.T46   2001   152.4—dc21   00-054849

For Leah and Kara,
  two loved ones who provided support for me in writing this book.

Contents

Preface

Alarming predictions about the epidemic of obesity have been the subject of countless discussions in the popular media, fueled by dire warnings from public health experts. But the reasons why so many more people are overweight or obese have remained mysterious. Why we eat too much and exercise too little becomes apparent when we look at mood as the backdrop of our lives. Much of what we do, day in and day out, revolves around our moods and the ways we attempt to manage them. Society at large provides an important stage for our mood-regulating activities. We live in a faster-paced and more stressful world than our grandparents did. Many people turn to food as a kind of self-medication.

In this book I try to clarify the active role our complicated moods play in our daily lives, including how we experience energy and tension. I try to show that poor eating habits and the avoidance of exercise are directly traceable to these moods. I also demonstrate how our awareness of important signals provided by our bodies can be effectively used to manage overeating and to increase exercise.

This book is not a self-help manual, but I do try to provide clear suggestions about how to control overeating and how to motivate ourselves to exercise. Since I started my scientific studies, over two decades ago, I have had an abiding interest in the nature of mood and in what causes our moods to change. My first research projects took place in the physiological laboratory with precise experimental manipulations and observations, but later they progressed to a naturalistic setting with analyses of how moods affect the totality of our lives. Throughout the years, I have seen how food and exercise are central to mood change, but the exact evidence for these interrelationships has remained maddeningly elusive until relatively recently. The latest scientific research has finally made these connections clear. I dealt with the theoretical issues of this topic in my previous books, *The Origin of Everyday Moods* and *The Biopsychology of Mood and Arousal,* but here I give full attention to mood, food, and exercise; nowhere else have these dynamics been fully explained.

My ideas are based on solid scientific research, presented in clearly understandable language. The field of weight control and exercise maintenance has become overrun with hype. In this book I steer clear of the oversimplification and unscientific claims of so many publications on diet and exercise, with the result, I hope, that readers will come away informed and enlightened.

Many people have been helpful in the creation of this book, not the least of which are the students in my university classes, who have analyzed and followed in detail the variations of mood and its influence on food and exercise. I have learned a great deal from these discussions, and frequently I realized I was going in the wrong direction in my thinking when practical examples were fleshed out in class discussions. It is extraordinarily helpful for a researcher to have a group of such thoughtful and educated people to consider ideas and offer suggestions.

In addition to this general help, I am particularly thankful to students, colleagues, and friends whose cases I use to clarify concepts in this book. Sometimes I have kept their real names; in other cases the names and insignificant life details were changed to maintain anonymity; in a couple of cases the experiences of two or more people were combined to make a point.

Of the individuals who helped me in writing this book, none was more important than Joan Bossert, my editor at Oxford University Press. She not only supported and encouraged my pursuit of these matters at early stages but also read, critiqued, and offered suggestions, chapter by chapter. Repeatedly, I was struck by her understanding and insights into technical psychological concepts, which seemed on many occasions on a par with those of my colleagues who are scientists. And, expert as she is in principles of good communication in print, she was able to call my attention to places where I strayed off course and often to suggest ways to get back on track.

I wish especially to thank Retha Evans, who patiently read and commented on each chapter. She often gave me the confidence I needed to know I was on the right track. And, sorting expertly through the complex concepts involved, she would go straight to the core of the matter in her analyses of my writing and facts as I presented them.

I would also like to thank three well-known scientists who read portions of the book and made many helpful comments. The distinguished physiological psychologist Alexander Beckman provided excellent observations and suggestions about the physiology discussed in the book. Larry Christensen, recognized widely for his important research and writing on diet and behavior, offered good ideas for parts of the book. And Steven Petruzzello, an exercise scientist whose outstanding research is widely recognized, provided many important suggestions. Since these scientists made suggestions that I did not always follow, I am to blame for any errors within.

Long Beach, California   R.E.T.

Calm Energy

CHAPTER 1

Mood, Self-Regulation, and Overeating

YOUR MOODS DETERMINE your enjoyment of life. When you are in a good mood, enjoyable activities can be great fun, even exciting. You deal with the things you put off, though you find them unpleasant. But when you are anxious, you feel like snapping at everyone. You probably feel irritable, and you may even develop depression. The world looks dark and uninviting, and everything seems hopeless. It doesn't matter how often people tell you that things are fine; a negative cast to all the events that take place in your life clouds your ability to enjoy simple pleasures. In a very real sense your moods are more important than events, since your moods determine how much of those events you will be able to enjoy.

Your mood systems, as we sometimes refer to them scientifically, reflect your physical as well as your psychological being. If you ask the average person what causes moods, you will often get an answer that is only partially right. He or she will tell you that events and circumstances control our moods: "He was rude to me"; "My car broke down"; "I had trouble at work." But if you think logically about this, you will see that there is a problem with it. Events and circumstances are often random, but our moods are closely related to how much sleep we had, how healthy we are, when and what we last ate, and what kind of exercise we had lately. Even the time of day is important to our moods.

Furthermore, our moods are correlated with the momentary biochemical reactions of our brain: our hormones coursing through our bodies in differing concentrations at one time or another, blood sugar levels in continuous variation, the tension of our muscles rapidly changing as we encounter problems or feel relaxed, and a host of other shifting physiological reactions. Moods change, and we can identify the biological conditions that are the most probable underpinnings of those changes.[1] Events and circumstances do influence mood, but they happen on top of a biological edifice that gives them greater or lesser importance.

For well over two decades I have studied these issues as a scientist, and one of the most interesting findings that consistently emerges concerns how people try to *self-regulate* their moods. I find that this is almost like a self-medication process. The list of things we use to control our moods and feelings from moment to moment is endless: food, drink, social interaction, music, coffee, cigarettes, intentionally diverting our thoughts, and much more. The behavior or substance we turn to can be thought of as something like a drug of choice. We all want to avoid bad moods, and we all want to be in a good mood as much as possible.

Research has shown again and again that we are constantly self-regulating our mood.[2] Sometimes it is conscious, but often we aren't aware that we are relying on certain habits to accomplish this, habits we resort to when we are feeling slightly out of sorts. We all do things to make ourselves feel good, and when we are feeling bad (a bad mood) we turn to those things that worked in the past. Much of the time, our methods of self-control work very well, but some of the things we use to self-regulate work only temporarily and leave us in a worse mood in the long run. Chris is an example of someone using a method successfully.

Chris, a returning college student in her early forties, seems to know how to control her moods, at least for a while. When she is in a bad mood, she immediately calls one of three good friends. They all have more or less the same mood-regulating strategy, like the women in the movie *The First Wives Club*. They arrange lunch or a trip to the mall for some shopping, and Chris says it works. At the end of the lunch, or after an afternoon at the mall, she feels good again. Those mild but annoying feelings of depression have vanished.

In one extensive set of studies about ways that people self-regulate their moods, we found that, when bad moods occur, the first thing most people do is to seek some kind of social interaction.[3] They pick up the phone. Or they try to be with someone, especially someone who will listen to them and make them feel better. Women are much more likely to do this than men, but both sexes do it.[4] When a bad mood becomes obvious, another common thing that we found people doing is to try to change the way they are thinking. They try to think positively, or to think about something other than their troublesome problem. They also try not to let things bother them. Many people give themselves a pep talk when their mood is low. Men use these cognitive techniques more than women, but again it's a strategy that both sexes use.

When our mood is low, almost half of us listen to music to regulate our feelings. Younger people listen to music more than others. My daughter Leah is a good example. She has a whole library of CDs and tapes that she listens to selectively, depending on her mood. When I told her about the results of our research showing how often people use music for mood regulation, she wasn't at all surprised.

Older people turn, instead, to other routines that make them feel better. They may tend to their chores—cleaning the house, working in the garden, catching up on correspondence. These appear to be excellent mood regulators. My late mother was always in a good mood. She had certain healthy routines that probably contributed to her positive disposition. For example, in a typical day she would work on her garden in the morning, then she would straighten up the house and go to the market. Later she'd write letters or read spiritual books of interest to her. This last practice is especially consistent with our research findings. Many older people told us that they turn to religious and spiritual activities as a way of feeling better when their mood is low. Social scientists often lose sight of how seemingly mundane daily activities like chores or gardening, and spiritual activities such as regular religious observances and prayer, can have strong influences on our mood.

About a third of us exercise when our moods are low.[5] This is a surprisingly small percentage, considering, as we will see in subsequent chapters, that moderate exercise is the best technique for feeling better immediately. It is effective, swift, and reliable. All of the things I mentioned work to raise our moods, but some, like exercise, work better than others.

Eating and Other Mood Regulators

About a third of us admit to eating as a way of self-regulating mood. Women admit this more than men do, but nearly everyone uses this method, at least from time to time.[6] No mystery here: eating good-tasting food makes us feel better right away. But a short time after we eat a sugary snack, our mood sinks (just sixty minutes later in one study).[7] Why do we eat when we really aren't hungry, when it breaks our diet and makes us feel bad about ourselves? The pleasure of eating is highly motivating, and the immediate good feeling it gives us is a lure. Even an overeater who regrets eating junk food and feels guilty soon after, or who feels tired and tense sixty minutes later, is controlled by her eating habit. In the psychology of learning, this is the well-known principle of positive reinforcement.[8]

Justine is a good example of someone who uses food to self-medicate. Most people who know her do not realize that she uses food this way because they never see her eating in public. But her weight gives away her mood-regulating habit. A young, fairly active woman, Justine is forty pounds overweight. Food, often consumed in private, is the primary way she regulates her mood.

For Mark, alcohol is the drug of choice. A few drinks with friends several times a week became drinks every night in front of the TV, then covert drinking during the day. Men are more likely than women to use alcohol to self-regulate their moods, but, once again, both sexes do turn to it.

For many people, cigarettes are continuous mood regulators and the nicotine habit is closely linked to a specific time interval. A person who smokes one to two packs a day lights up a cigarette every half-hour or so. When he finds himself in a meeting or someplace where he can't smoke, he will feel tense until he can smoke again. The tension will be apparent in his increasingly agitated demeanor. When left without a cigarette, addicted smokers are driven to avoid the unpleasant tension that builds. Their people mood regulation operates openly and continuously. The cigarette calms them down, gives them a lift, or, more often, does both.

Coffee, and caffeine in general, is another widely used mood regulator in our culture. Caffeine and tobacco work on our moods in a similar way that food does. Countless people depend on coffee and caffeinated soft drinks to feel better, not just in the morning to wake up. They drink it all day. (Just look at the success of Starbucks and other coffee bars.) Americans are hooked in this respect, and so are Europeans. One of my colleagues, a professor from Stockholm, told me that it isn't unusual for Swedes—who live in more northern latitudes than most people in this country—to ingest over 1000 milligrams of caffeine a day (that's more than ten cups of coffee). Of course, North Americans are not immune; a friend of mine suggested it is understandable why Starbucks originated in the northern city of Seattle, Washington.

Most of the time we aren't even aware of what we are doing when we try to control our moods. Habits are like that. If eating worked for us before, for example, when we feel bad, we develop a certain pattern without realizing it. First, our thoughts about good-tasting food begin to dominate our thinking, and it is a short step from thoughts to action. Of course, we may be reminded about a diet, and we know we shouldn't eat the forbidden food, but people have great powers of rationalization. "I didn't eat much last meal," we may tell ourselves, or "I deserve something good." Our excuses flow into mind with perfect ease. Even if we recognize these flimsy excuses for what they are, there often comes a point when we must eat the forbidden food because it is the only thing that will interrupt the urgency of the negative mood, even if just for a little while. Habits that worked before become almost automatic. They control us even in the face of strong resolve.

We regulate our mood when we feel bad, but we also do things to feel better when we are already feeling okay. We may overeat at a party or during pleasant interactions with our family and friends. Having a glass of wine with dinner or a cigarette when you feel contented are other good examples. Recreational drug users probably fall into this category. Others use exercise as a way of "firing up," as one of my students called it. She exercises when she wants to feel really good, not just all right. Here we aren't trying to escape from a bad feeling, but a kind of memory of things past that made us feel good now motivates us to reestablish that good mood once again.

When it comes to overeating, though, more often it is a negative mood that leads to it—"emotional eating," many people call it. This kind of mood regulation is the most important cause of overweight. In this book I concentrate on eating to change a bad mood, but I will come back to other kinds of positive self-regulation later, especially when we analyze the most optimal moods.

Mood and Overeating

In discussing overeating, countless magazine articles and popular books focus on the type and balance of foods you should eat, artificial appetite suppressants, natural metabolism differences, genetic predispositions, setpoint theory, and a host of variations. But managing your mood is one of the most important keys to controlling overeating. Most of the commonly discussed causes of overeating affect us through the mechanism of mood, in my view. For example, most scientists today accept the fact that there are genetic predispositions to overweight, but exactly how this occurs is not understood. I suggest that one likely causal path is through the food and mood link.

On the topic of food and mood, there is a body of credible evidence, but it is not about how different foods affect our moods—there is not as much reliable evidence about that. Instead, it is about how our moods affect our desire to eat. In one review of more than fifty scientific studies of emotional eating, the triggering emotions or moods invariably were identified as depression, anxiety, anger, boredom, and loneliness.[9] Most studies focus on the way these negative moods occur immediately before a diet is broken or as a likely cause of some eating disorder, including obesity. In my view, if you forget everything else—including the kinds of food to eat, their relative proportions and exact amounts—but you master your moods, you will go a long way toward controlling overeating.[10]

Although negative moods control our eating because good-tasting food allows us to counteract these unpleasant feelings, this relationship is more complicated than it appears. We know that bad moods are characterized by low energy and good moods with high energy. For example, when you are feeling depressed you have little energy, but in the best moods your energy is abundant. Food offers an immediate correction for low energy; it relieves your tension and gives you a lift. We may not think of food as an energy enhancer, but that is its effect. If you doubt that food energizes you, notice sometime when you are driving while tired—an unwise thing to do—that eating a snack wakes you up a little. It allows you to stay alert, even if only for a little while.[11] (Incidentally, if you eat a lot of rich food, you may wake up for a little while, but soon you can expect to feel even more tired.)[12] When we feel better after we eat, it is partly from this elevated energy.

A Theory of What Moods Tell Us

Negative moods are like subtle indications that we need more energy. When we self-regulate our moods to make ourselves feel better, we raise our energy. We react to our moods at some level of consciousness, however deep. Therefore, these moods subtly guide our decisions and actions with regard to food, a ready energy source.[13] This guidance in the form of motivation to eat is not always immediate, but over time it has an effect. One of the best indications of the energy-food link is that overeating typically occurs when energy is low. That is one reason diets are most often broken in the late afternoon and evening, times of lower energy. I believe that motivation to eat something to raise our energy when our moods are low is a basic biological response.

Tense or anxious moods, which often prompt us to eat, are also signals of a need for more energy—in this case, the energy necessary to overcome adversity.[14] When you are energized, even a dangerous situation can be at least tolerable. In addition, stress often is a stimulus for eating poorly, as we shall see in later chapters. And depression that is characterized by elevated tension as well as low energy is clearly associated with eating problems, including bulimia and other kinds of bingeing.[15]

Tension is important to eating in another way. When we diet and try to avoid eating a tempting food, a small amount of tension results. In biological terms, tension is a basic part of inhibitory and cautious behaviors (we sometimes speak of a bodily "stop system").[16] It is an indication in our consciousness that we must be on guard. Dieting requires vigilance—both to withstand the craving for good-tasting but unnecessary food and to manage your lifestyle in such a way as to continue the diet. I will deal with these ideas much more fully in later chapters, but from these points I aim to establish my argument that both tension and energy are important elements of mood and that we often use food to achieve a positive mood.

A Personal Example of How Moods Cause Overeating

A while ago I went to the airport to pick up my daughter Kara, who was flying into Los Angeles from northern California. It was about 5:00 P.M., and I had eaten a late lunch—light but nutritious. As I watched the flight information board, a message appeared that her plane had been diverted. Anxiety immediately gripped me. The gate attendant told the people waiting that the plane had to make an unscheduled landing in Fresno, but she assured us that it must be only a minor problem. Regardless of what she said, these were anxious moments for me and the dozens of other people who were waiting for loved ones on the plane. Thirty minutes later we learned that there had been a medical emergency and that the plane landed briefly to let off a passenger. We were assured that the plane had taken off again and would be there shortly.

As I relaxed some of my concerns, I felt slightly drained (low energy) and suddenly noticed I was hungry. The convenience stand nearby caught my eye with its rows of candy bars neatly lined up. I bought a Snickers and a Diet Coke and consumed them with pleasure. Generally, I avoid excessive sugar and fat, and I try to keep my intake of caffeine to a small amount. This time I wanted the sugar and the caffeine because I knew it would counteract the unpleasant drained and tense feeling and make me feel better for my daughter's arrival. As I made a decision to buy the candy and soda, I thought about the fact that I didn't really need them, but I quickly rationalized the matter with some vague excuse about deserving it.

When I thought about this incident later, it was clear that when I first saw the sign about the plane being diverted, I wasn't hungry at all. I was too anxious. But when the worst was over, and there was still a little tension mixed with a drained or low energy feeling, my desire for sugar and caffeine overcame my normal inhibitions against eating these things. My indulgence was a way of regulating my mood, albeit a temporary one. Incidentally, the relationship between different intensities of mood and eating in this example is instructive for self-understanding: high anxiety or tension often reduces eating, but low-level anxiety, particularly tension combined with low energy, often increases it.[17] Knowing this can enable you to understand and get control over many unwanted food urges.

How We Regulate Our Energy

In our daily lives we control and self-regulate our energy in many different ways. Dead-tired in the morning, we still get up and move around, and through this physical activity we feel more energetic. Activity wakes us up, and it is a kind of self-regulation. Or we use a substance like coffee to energize ourselves. Snacking is another way that we control our energy from moment to moment. We eat to regulate ourselves, both to counteract our negative moods and to keep ourselves going, to keep ourselves alert and energetic. And sometimes we eat to make ourselves feel good, even though we don't feel particularly bad at the time.

Consider an example in which you are sitting at home watching television. The program is boring, and you find yourself getting tired. But it isn't time for bed yet, so your thoughts turn to the Oreos in the kitchen. Your energy surges slightly as you think how good they would taste. This is a conditioned reaction, learned from snacking in the past. But you don't succumb immediately. Perhaps you turn again to the boring program. Then the thoughts return, and eventually you go into the kitchen with a resolve to eat just one cookie. But, the single cookie activates your taste for more, and since you already have overcome your resolve to avoid the sweets, you eat several.[18] (It is hard to stop at just one cookie, and the conditioning is so strong that many people can't stop before they've eaten a whole box.)[19] What I am talking about here are momentary impulses that really have to do with subtle changes in your energy and tension levels. These short-term feelings or moods can control us if we aren't careful. Understanding the way they operate is crucial to gaining self-control.

Self-Control

If we could feel better in some other, more healthy, way than eating junk food, we wouldn't eat unnecessarily.[20] The management of unwanted urges to eat is really a matter of controlling our negative moods, especially the momentary ones. If you think of the cause of overeating in this way, it becomes obvious that becoming aware of the subtle influences of our negative moods, and changing them, can correct our overeating. Scientists have discovered lots of reasons for overeating and obesity, but in my view mood is a vital link.

Can overeating be controlled so it isn't a life-long problem? The answer is yes. Awareness of what is happening, and that means understanding the way our moods control our eating habits, is much of the battle. When food is no longer used as a mood regulator, then normal appetite will regulate our intake. When our physical resources decline and we need sustenance, we become hungry. When we have had enough food for the immediate demands of our body, we stop eating. It's a marvelous system that our biology provides. Evolution has honed our bodies into smooth-running systems. Appetite isn't our enemy. It tells us exactly what we need.

Negative moods tell us what we need as well. But they tell us that we need energy. This reaction is probably honed over eons from a precarious environment of predators and inadequate food supplies. Our ancestors had to react appropriately or they didn't survive, and negative moods represented important information in that survival process. We are the descendants of the survivors. Because food is the most easily obtainable source of energy, we often turn to it. Thus, the motivation to eat when our moods are low is perfectly understandable. Take negative moods away and normal bodily needs govern our appetite and the amount that we eat. It seems too simple, but it is true.

In the pages that follow, we will examine negative moods, including when they motivate overeating and when they do not. And we will see what can be done to manage the negative moods that impel us to eat. We explore how positive or optimal moods can be maintained, and how these states lead not only to healthy reactions to food but to a host of other ingredients of a pleasurable life.

Mood and Lack of Exercise

Why we overeat is a main theme of this book. Another important theme is why we don't exercise enough. And as we will see, our moods once again have a fundamental motivational role, in this case leading to the tendency to avoid physical activity. So the same moods that drive us to overeat inhibit the very exercise that we need to prevent overweight. And the process of self-regulation of moods that we understand in relation to overeating applies as well to lack of exercise. But the predominant mood states that often result in overeating, including stress reactions and depression, involve lack of energy and tension, and these states motivate us in the short run to remain inactive, to rest, or to sleep.

We will see that this tendency to become inactive when we feel depressed is ironic because one of the very best ways of counteracting depression is to exercise. In the pages that follow we will examine some of the reasons why moods inhibit exercise and also how our understanding of this tendency can be used to counteract the tendency to be inactive.

A Look Ahead

In the next chapter I will examine the problem of overeating and unhealthy weight. As we will see, millions of people in our society are engaged on a daily basis in the struggle to control their weight. It has become a national obsession, and a battle we seem to be losing. Why? I will argue that certain conditions in our society create mood states that motivate many of us to eat unnecessarily. Developing trends, especially in the past twenty or thirty years, determine these tendencies for overweight and indolence. In the third chapter I will deal with the way exercise affects eating, overweight, and mood, and also with the question of why people aren't exercising more.

Chapters 4 and 5 will carefully examine the now abundant scientific studies of how moods cause overeating. In these chapters we will also consider the subtle relationship between exercise and eating, including the often competing pleasure and energy functions that the two provide. The next three chapters will be a more complete examination of moods—how they work, what causes them, and the underlying biology. Finally, we will consider some ways of managing moods and thus how to deal with the problems of overeating and lack of exercise.

CHAPTER 2

Living in a Stressful World

Mood and Overweight

O BESITY HAS BECOME a national problem. The statistics on this matter are clear: we are becoming a nation of fatties. This change has been especially evident since the 1980s. Although the experts don't agree on the reason for the overeating and overweight, it is clear that basic issues of food, mood, and lack of exercise extend throughout society. A wider lens focusing on societal trends that may affect eating and exercise can illustrate many of the principles touched on in Chapter 1, here applied to millions of people.

Two trends that might be contributing to overweight and lack of exercise are stress and depression, both on the upswing. Before reviewing these trends, let's pause to determine whether overweight is really a concern throughout society—or just a hype that sells books and newspapers.

Is Overweight a Society-Wide Problem?

Some suggest that descriptions of increasing obesity are exaggerated, but the fact is that between half and two-thirds of American adults report being overweight in poll after poll, and these figures have been creeping up in recent years.[1] Systematic telephone surveys by the Center for Disease Control and Prevention found that obesity (defined as 30 percent above ideal body weight) increased by almost 50 percent between 1991 and 1998.[2] If anything, these figures underestimate the prevalence of obesity, because most people believe (or report) their weight to be lower than it actually is. Look around and see how many people appear over-weight and you can begin to sense the truth about obesity.

These statistics are astounding. Obesity increased in both men and women in all age groups—and since those between the ages of eighteen to twenty-nine gained the most, it isn't just that the population is aging. Some of the greatest increases showed up among those with more educa-tion. States in the Mid- and South Atlantic region marked the largest change, but the obesity epidemic is apparent throughout the country. And the weight gains occurred with no substantial change in physical activity.

The rise in obesity itself no doubt contributes to many people's exces-sive concerns about their weight. In one *Psychology Today* survey of read-ers, 24 percent of women said they would sacrifice more than three years of their lives to be the weight they want![3] Earlier surveys by the same magazine did not show this degree of distress about weight. Other people have stopped being concerned about their increasing weight, arguing heredity—as though they have no personal responsibility because their genes completely determine their weight.[4] This is a misreading of the sci-entific evidence about our genetic endowment. While our genetic back-ground can create a *predisposition* for easy weight gain,[5] this only means that some people must be especially vigilant about how much they eat and exercise. It does not mean that they definitely will be overweight.[6] In any event, our collective genetic background is not changing so dramatically as to account for the changes in obesity observed in the last two decades. If these changes are in fact occurring, something else must be propelling them.

Is it possible that people are incorrectly perceiving their degree of overweight, and that the percentage of obese people has not grown much? Could it just be a neurotic society-wide preoccupation? Alas, the answer is no. The larger trend is unmistakable. One of our most authoritative sci-entific journals, *Science*, recently devoted extensive scientific analyses to the problem of overweight, and the conclusions by highly respected scien-tists made it clear that Americans have been gaining weight steadily in the last twenty years or so.[7] This weight increase has alarmed many health professionals. Former U.S. Surgeon General C. Everett Koop, for exam-ple, declared an epidemic of obesity not just in the United States but around the world as well.[8]

Back in the 1950s the well-known Metropolitan Life Insurance Com-

BODY MASS INDEX

Height \ Weight	100	105	110	115	120	125	130	135	140	145	150	155	160	165	170	175	180	185	190	195	200	205
5'0"	20	21	21	22	23	24	25	26	27	28	29	30	31	32	33	34	35	36	37	38	39	40
5'1"	19	20	21	22	23	24	25	26	26	27	28	29	30	31	32	33	34	35	36	37	38	39
5'2"	18	19	20	21	22	23	24	25	26	27	27	28	29	30	31	32	33	34	35	36	37	37
5'3"	18	19	19	20	21	22	23	24	25	26	27	27	28	29	30	31	32	33	34	35	35	36
5'4"	17	18	19	20	21	21	22	23	24	25	26	27	27	28	29	30	31	32	33	33	34	35
5'5"	17	17	18	19	20	21	22	22	23	24	25	26	27	27	28	29	30	31	32	32	33	34
5'6"	16	17	18	19	19	20	21	22	23	23	24	25	26	27	27	28	29	30	31	31	32	33
5'7"	16	16	17	18	19	20	20	21	22	23	23	24	25	26	27	27	28	29	30	31	31	32
5'8"	15	16	17	17	18	19	20	21	21	22	23	24	24	26	26	27	27	28	29	30	30	31
5'9"	15	16	16	17	18	18	19	20	21	21	22	23	24	24	25	26	27	27	28	29	30	31
5'10"	14	15	16	17	17	18	19	19	20	21	22	22	23	24	24	25	26	27	27	28	29	29
5'11"	14	15	15	16	17	17	18	19	20	20	21	22	22	23	24	24	25	26	26	27	28	29
6'0"	14	14	15	16	16	17	18	18	19	20	20	21	22	22	23	24	24	25	26	26	27	28
6'1"	13	14	15	15	16	16	17	18	18	19	20	20	21	22	22	23	24	24	25	26	26	27
6'2"	13	13	14	15	15	16	17	17	18	19	19	20	21	21	22	22	23	24	24	25	26	26
6'3"	12	13	14	14	15	16	16	17	17	18	19	19	20	21	21	22	22	23	24	24	25	26
6'4"	12	13	13	14	15	15	16	16	17	18	18	19	19	20	21	21	22	23	23	24	24	25

Where do you stand? This chart shows how BMIs (numbers in squares) vary with weight and height. Some think that BMIs of 26 to 27 carry moderate health risks, with risks increasing further as BMIs rise.

pany tables were the standard that determined appropriate weight according to one's age and sex. We now know that these standards were rather lax and they have been replaced by the more precise Body Mass Index (BMI), which is an indication of the amount of body fat.[9] But the observation that we are gaining weight isn't based just on this more rigorous standard. People are actually getting fatter.[10]

Some scientists wonder whether it is because fewer people smoke, a habit that tends to control weight. Or is it because of the easy abundance of energy-intensive junk food, or increased sedentariness? Each of these explanations is a possibility, but none seems likely to account for the big changes observed.

Then there is the issue of whether this overweight really is a problem. But as an answer to this, we can point to a number of large-scale studies that show correlations between overweight and various disorders, especially cardiovascular heart disease. Often cited as evidence of this relationship are such studies as the famous Framingham Heart Study, conducted in Framingham, Massachusetts, where over 5,000 people were examined in 1949 and then followed up twenty-six years later.[11] High weight predicted cardiovascular heart disease, particularly among women. Confirming these results were later studies such as the so-called Nurses Health Study of over 115,000 female nurses, which showed that body weight and mortality from all causes were directly related among middle-aged women.[12] More recently, a study of over 300,000 men and women showed that Body Mass Index was associated with higher mortality from all causes, at least up to seventy-five years of age.[13] Interestingly, this study found that the risk from increased body weight was greater among younger persons. Other studies confirm that overweight and obesity substantially contribute to chronic health conditions.[14]

But is mere overweight the problem, or do these associations with increased mortality occur because overweight people are not usually fit? Steven Blair and his colleagues at the Cooper Institute for Aerobics Research argue that fitness is a critical predictor.[15] In a recent 1998 PBS *Frontline* special entitled *Fat*, fifty-nine-year-old Blair, who could be categorized as clinically obese, was featured running as part of his weekly regimen of 35 miles. Short, stocky, and very fit, Blair argues that his body type, which conserves body mass and would allow him to survive a famine, might be similar to that of a hardy serf in the Russian Steppes and could be quite adaptive from an evolutionary perspective.

Health risks aside, most sophisticated social observers realize that perceptions about overweight are based to some extent on cultural fashions rather than health. A lot of people seem awfully concerned about having a little extra weight. In time of famine, after all, overweight people would be better equipped to survive than their skinny counterparts, and this is a kind of big-picture biological proof that overweight isn't all that bad. Fashions change, as we know. Women who were considered beautiful like Marilyn Monroe and Mae West—earlier this century—look downright heavy to us now.

Without making a judgment about how important obesity is, we can try to understand the influences that could produce it. Assuming that obesity, as judged by current standards, is a growing problem, are there trends in society that could be contributing to it? I argue that an important influence can be found in the undeniable fact that our collective mood is worsening, as evidenced by the increasing incidence of stress and depression and related disorders. I believe that negative moods induce people to self-regulate in order to correct the problem. This means greater reliance on food, among other things, as a mood-altering substance.

Is Stress Increasing in Society?

At twenty-nine years, Mike has begun to achieve tangible success in his sales specialty. But this has been at some cost. His girlfriend hardly ever sees him. Often the only way she can reach him is on his cell phone, or they exchange hurried voice-mail messages. When they finally make contact at night, he is usually very tired, and probably because of this they have sex only about once a month. He complains continually about not having enough time.

Although Mike was very athletic in his younger years, his body is starting to deteriorate and his gut is growing unpleasantly large. Obesity is becoming a real problem for him, just as it was for his father and his older brothers. His genes predispose him to easy weight gain, so he has to be especially vigilant not to succumb to that predicament. Instead he is doing all the wrong things.

Mike's immediate problem is stress and lack of time. He eats only on the run. Fast-food drive-throughs have become his restaurants of choice. They allow him to pop in between appointments for a quick, good-tasting meal that gives him an immediate energy surge. He is in the car much of the time, where he always keeps a supply of doughnuts or muffins and a big container of coffee to pick himself up when he is hit by the inevitable postmeal slump. He drives everywhere rather than walking—he just doesn't have time—and his regular exercise routine is long gone. He ingests many more calories than his on-the-go lifestyle uses up.

Our society is filled with Mikes, for whom stress is an ever-present condition. Their tension is high and their energy resources are often drained. As they desperately try to right themselves through an elemental kind of self-regulation with food, their eating habits deteriorate and they seek the most energy-intensive foods. Is it any wonder that obesity is on the rise?

Public opinion polls can give us some reliable information about levels of stress and about trends. For example, in the 1980s many public opinion polls asked a standard question, or some close variation of it: "How often are you under great stress?"[16] On average, 14.4 percent of respondents said they were under stress every day. In the 1990s that figure had risen to 18.1 percent.[17] The increase holds true for younger as well as older people. And women appear to be under greater stress than men.[18] Could this be why women suffer more from problems of over-weight than men do—self-regulating with food in an effort to reduce stress?

What Is the Cause of Increasing Societal Stress?

American society and other societies the world over are experiencing an ever-increasing pace of life. In 1970 Alvin Toffler published an influential and best-selling book titled *Future Shock*, which startled people into sudden awareness that we were increasing stress and reshaped our thinking about forced change.[19] He warned that in three short decades, between then and now, millions of people would face what he called an abrupt collision with the future. He showed how this change was beginning even then, as reflected in the products people bought, the communities they lived in, the organizations they belonged to, the mass media that bombarded them, and even in their friendships and love. They were shocking when we read about them back in the 1970s, but all of Toffler's predictions about the future have already taken place.

In his 1999 book, *Faster: The Acceleration of Just About Everything*, James Glick excellently portrays our rapid pace: "If one quality defines our modern, technological age, it is acceleration. We are making haste. Our computers, our movies, our sex lives, our prayers – they all run faster now than ever before. And the more we fill our lives with time-saving devices and time-saving strategies, the more rushed we feel."[20]

Sometimes it's difficult to see change when you are in the midst of it. But consider a simple example that illustrates the changes that have taken place in the last two decades. Those who are old enough will remember a time when going to the movies meant going to a double feature and sitting there for three or four hours. Can you imagine a large number of modern-day people now spending their time in this way? If you think the pace of life hasn't become more speeded, take a few hours to watch some early sitcoms that are being recycled on cable TV. You can't help but notice their slow pace. People liked it then, but today we would insist on more action, quicker pace, getting to the point faster. Life has sped up and it is affecting us in many ways, not the least of which is our overall mood and how we try to regulate it.

Public opinion polls clearly indicate that time is a problem for many people. Moreover, the pressure that comes from feeling that there is too little time is increasing. For example, fifteen years ago 18 percent of respondents thought that lack of time was a source of much stress in relationships between husbands and wives.[21] But less than ten years later, 28 percent believed that time pressure was a major cause of stress.[22] And more recently, 30 percent reported that the demands on their time represented a lot of stress for them.[23]

Juggling Commitments of Work and Family

Mary, a thirty-five-year-old middle executive, is divorced and lives alone with her child. She balances her responsibilities to Cory, her eight-year-old, with a demanding job that takes most of her energy to do well. Her mom didn't have these demands. She only had Mary and her sister to look after. And her dad, the major breadwinner, wasn't concerned, as Mary is, about his company downsizing.

To keep her job secure, Mary works long hours. At the end of each day, she is exhausted. What little energy she has left, she tries to spend on Cory, who passes much of her day at school and in an after-hours child-care facility. Mary doesn't have the kind of built-in social support that many couples use to elevate their mood. In the five years since her divorce, she has gained thirty pounds. Mary's main way of regulating her mood, especially at night, is to eat. She hates herself for doing it, but food is her only reliable solace and source of pleasure. No matter how much she promises herself at the high times of her day that she will maintain a strict diet, she can't resist snacking when her energy drops. Good-tasting food is like a drug, and Mary is like an addict.

Books, newspaper articles, and radio and TV programs often identify work as a major source of stress. This is a time of dual-income families, longer hours spent on the job, and more time spent on the road. Bruce Kaufman, an economics professor at Georgia State University, summed up the current conditions in this way: "We try to sandwich everything into our lives to be good employees, be good parents, be good citizens, get everything done, all in twenty-four hours a day, and the demand is just too much."[25]

A *National Public Radio* special recently described the prevailing situation, especially as it impacts women, by saying that this is a time of great economic change within the work place with changing expectations of men and women playing a large role in our society's new work ethic.[25] Moreover, as men and women are doing similar tasks at home and at work, there is much more to reach agreement about. Indeed, juggling work and home schedules probably makes women's lives even more stressful than men's.

Downsizing is a continuous source of stress. Even though employment may be high, workers are always looking over their shoulders about what is to come. An International Survey Research poll recently found that 44 percent of those polled worry frequently about being laid off—a substantial increase from the 22 percent who worried about it in 1988.[26] In a recent Gallup poll, eight in ten respondents described themselves as overworked and stressed out as a result of years of downsizing.[27] People are working more hours just to keep up—an average of 44 hours a week, up from 40 hours a week in 1989.[28]

Another change in the workplace that has produced increased stress is the rapid rise in temp work. A recent *Los Angeles Times* analysis of this phenomenon described how companies increasingly are turning to this form of hiring because, by keeping their workforce temporary, companies can control payroll and production costs according to immediate demand. But as the article points out, "In this jittery new world, a layoff is simply an 'end of assignment,' job security is unknown, and most of the risk of fluctuating markets is transferred from employer to employee."[29] Previous temp workers mainly were clerical, but industrial workers almost have caught up in numbers. While good for the bottom line of companies, temp work is inherently stressful for the worker.

Steve Sauter, the primary author of *Stress at Work*, a new report by the National Institute of Occupational Safety and Health, puts it well: "The issue is the feeling of having no control over rapid change and job security."[30] A strong indication that stress and the accompanying tension are on the rise can be seen in the fact that absenteeism has gone up 25 percent in seven years, according to a survey of 401 executives of U.S. organizations of all sizes. This survey revealed that most sick days involve stress-related issues, including job fatigue, as well as taking care of aging parents and sick children. [31]

This rise in stress and tension is clear when you compare recent public opinion polls with those taken a decade earlier. A 1998 Gallup poll found that 45 percent of adults are bothered by stress on their job at least several days a week (19 percent every day).[32] In a 1997 *Washington Post* poll 59 percent of respondents said work-related pressure contributes to stress at least somewhat often (20 percent very often).[33] And 73 percent of respondents in a Princeton Survey Research poll believe that there is more stress for the average working person compared to twenty or thirty years ago.[34] Compare these figures with those reported ten years earlier in the 1980s when stress was evident, but not the amount that we now experience. Between 1984 and 1987, for example, three national polls found that between 13 percent and 15 percent of respondents saw job demands as causing a great deal of stress—indications of high stress, but nothing like those evident just ten years later.[35]

Stress in the Information Age

Another significant source of stress is the information and communication explosion. Recently I listened to a talk given by Phillip Zimbardo, the psychologist from Stanford University, in which he described the change in social interaction and communication that has taken over his department: colleagues now sit in their offices and e-mail each other rather than walking down the hall to ask a question or to say something to a friend. At my university, office doors used to be open, but now they are closed. If you want to communicate, you must use e-mail or leave a voice mail or catch someone on a cell phone. I can remember when the excuse for a late paper was that a typewriter ribbon ran out. The excuse I am more likely to get today is that the computer crashed. Personal computers with all their astonishing complexity were hardly envisioned when Toffler wrote *Future Shock*, but they are a fact of life today. And today if an assignment is given that requires research, I am likely to hear excuses for late papers that involve problems logging onto the Internet. The databases of information available to students today through the Internet are almost overwhelming, and they would not have been believed only a few short years ago.

USA Today recently analyzed these new developments and referred to what they dubbed "techno stress."[36] In the business world, clients used to be content to wait a day or two for a letter to arrive, but now they want it faxed immediately. While these developments have increased productivity, they have a clear downside. Workers find that the new technology has made them devote too much time to sorting through electronic information and answering e-mail. Moreover, the new technology seduces employees into continuing work at home instead of taking a break. The pace of our lives is quickening, and it is taking its toll. Increased tension levels are the inevitable result.

How Do We Try to Counteract Stress?

How are people reacting to this growing negative pressure? One reaction has to do with poor food choices: in one poll, 45 percent of respondents indicated that stress caused them to have bad eating habits.[37] In another poll, 35 percent of respondents indicated that they sometimes eat to help relieve the stress in their daily life, and another 13 percent said they always eat to relieve stress.[38] Thus, almost half the population apparently uses food at least some of the time for stress relief. It is easy to see why. As tension rises, readily accessible energy foods are an easy antidote.

But what alternatives are there? Exercise is the single best remedy for bad moods—states characterized by increased tension and decreased energy.[39] And as stress has increased in society, some people do report that they exercise more.[40] But do most people exercise enough, given the dramatic increases in stress that are occurring? Absolutely not. Less than half of us use exercise to relieve stress. Everyone under stress should be exercising regularly. This is not to mention the positive effect that exercise has in controlling appetite for unnecessary foods (a matter that will be discussed more fully in Chapter 5).

Other ways of counteracting stress include talking on the telephone. In one Roper poll 27 percent of women reported often dealing with stress this way, but only 8 percent of men often did.[41] In our own research, we found that calling, talking to, or being with someone is one of the best ways of counteracting negative moods.[42] Men should take note—this is one lesson you can learn from women.

Listening to music is another great way to counteract a bad mood. Sleeping more can be helpful, too, if the negative state results from tiredness. As we shall see in later chapters of this book, people are sleeping fewer hours today than ever before. The resultant fatigue is surely one of the most important reasons why our collective mood is deteriorating.

Three other ways of dealing with stress have been reported in national polls. Forty-three percent of adults indicated that they often or sometimes work on a hobby when they are under stress.[43] In our study of moods we found that this is a very effective technique, perhaps because it takes people's minds off their problems and offers an enjoyable activity. We also found that this technique is used more by older people—perhaps through a kind of wisdom that comes with age. In another finding, we learned that many women use shopping as a mood elevator, and while the evidence was mixed on the effectiveness of this for the majority of people, some women found it very effective, and this may be because it often involves some moderate exercise and social interaction. In one national poll, 60 percent of women reported using shopping for stress relief at least sometimes (20 percent often), but only 30 percent of men use shopping for this purpose (6 percent often).[44] Finally, 75 percent of adults reported watching TV as a way of relieving stress. TV is one of the least effective ways of elevating mood.[45] Nonetheless, it is understandable how when drained of resources, many people cannot motivate themselves to do more than "vegetate" in front of the television. It clearly distracts them from thinking about their problems. But eating often accompanies this vegetative TV watching, and the inevitable outcome is weight gain.

A dramatic rise in stress has occurred in the past two decades, and we are trying to cope with the resulting tension and negative mood states as best we can. This escalating stress could underlie the increasing obesity that we see in society, but there is a second, and less known trend that may be equally important. This concerns the alarming increase in depression and related negative moods during the same twenty-year period. The added depression that mental health scientists are observing could be caused by stress, but that relationship is not clear. What is clear, however, is that overeating can be generated by some levels of depression, and, like stress, this could underlie the upsurge of obesity.

Depression: The Growing Epidemic

Elizabeth is forty-five. She was in a long-term marriage that she thought was secure, but her husband met a younger woman and left. She was already predisposed to negative moods through her genetic history—her grandmother had committed suicide and her mother was prone to pro-longed bouts of melancholy—and Elizabeth succumbed to a low-level depression that left her feeling tired most of the time. This fatigue was especially burdensome because her job demanded a great deal of her. As her boss would ask her to do more things, it was all she could do to avoid breaking down and crying.

During this time, her health habits deteriorated significantly. Although she maintained a membership in a health club, she stopped going. After coming home from work, she only had enough energy to fix herself a frozen dinner and flop down in front of the television for the rest of the evening. She started eating—and eating—until her body ballooned to unpleasant proportions. Food became her most reliable antidepressant, and one of the few sources of pleasure she had left.

But this case has a happy ending. Elizabeth finally got herself off the couch and went back to college to take some psychology classes. In a class of mine she learned about research showing how food, exercise, and mood are interrelated. The last time I talked to her she had reactivated her health club membership and joined the Sierra Club, which took her on frequent hikes. Her weight was dropping and her optimism was rising.

Many people, like Elizabeth, may be developing low-level depressions because they are continually under stress, a condition that makes them vul-nerable to psychological problems that do not bother people with higher levels of energy. Thus, Elizabeth's problem or a similar one could have a more profound effect than it would on a person who was more vigorous and hardy.[46] This could be one explanation for a huge increase in depression.

In the early 1980s a National Institute of Mental Health study sampled almost 20,000 Americans and found that a major depressive episode had occurred for 3.7 percent of adults in the preceding year, and for 6.4 per-cent at some point in their lives.[47] Ten years later those figures had risen to 10.3 percent and 17.1 percent—almost triple.[48] If *major* depressive episodes have increased to this degree in a ten-year period, it is highly likely that there has been an even greater increase in moderate depres-sion.[49] This is the kind of depression, for example, in which a person is only sometimes aware of even being depressed, or may not even identify the pervasive tiredness and lack of energy as depression.[50] In Chapter 4 we look at this kind of low-level depression as a factor that contributes to poor eating habits and obesity.

Tension-related disorders, such as panic attacks, are also on the rise. During the same ten-year period, there was an increase from 0.9 percent to 2.3 percent in these problems. In fact, in the 1990s study it was estimated that almost one in six adults (17.2 percent) had experienced some sort of anxiety disorder in the preceding year. Substance abuse, another indication of negative mood, showed comparable increases during that same period. (Incidentally, women experienced more depression and men experienced more substance abuse.)[51]

These psychological problems are not limited to adults. Recent headlines have revealed that childhood psychiatric emergencies are also on the rise, a trend that has been apparent for at least two decades.[52] A study at Yale University School of Medicine between 1995 and 1999 showed a 59 percent increase in admissions for depression, violence, drug ingestion, suicide attempts, and behavior changes among children ages four to fifteen. A report of a large-scale study involving thousands of children across the country recently released by the American Academy of Pediatrics showed that, in 1996, an alarming one out of five children had psychological or behavioral problems—twice as many as twenty years ago.[53] (Some might dismiss such increases as due to growing awareness and increased reporting by doctors, but the researchers took special care to evaluate that possibility and found it unlikely. For example, older doctors were just as likely to identify these problems as younger ones with more training in psychiatry.)

Public opinion polls taken from representative samples of all Americans clearly document this trend of increased depression and related disorders. A *Los Angeles Times* poll taken in 1989, for example, found that 9 percent of respondents reported that they were depressed fairly often or very often.[54] But by 1996, 15 percent reported they were very depressed at least about once a week, and another 14 percent said they were very depressed about once a month.[55] In a 1999 national poll, a full 21 percent of adult women said they have depression or an anxiety disorder.[56] Moreover, in that same survey 16 percent of women reported that they take antidepressant drugs, and another 17 percent said they had considered taking such drugs. Since there probably are many more people who are depressed than those taking antidepressants, these figures are astounding.[57] Depression and other psychological problems are clearly increasing at an alarming rate.

Are Depression and Stress
Linked to Problems with Overweight?

We live in a time when the value of exercise is widely assumed, when healthy and reduced-fat foods are readily available, when nutritional information has never been more accessible, yet obesity affects more people than ever. Why? I think it comes down to one thing: mood. Mood is central to our motivation both to eat and to avoid exercise.

The rampant stress and depression in our society can help us understand our motivation to eat more than we need and the lethargy we feel that exercise could allay. The mix of low energy and increased tension has never been experienced by so many people. Many of us try to cope by self-regulating our moods, too often by overeating or eating the wrong things.

Of course, not everyone reacts to negative conditions with increased eating. As we will see in subsequent chapters, the amount of stress and depression one feels can be an important determinant of whether he or she eats to feel better. Some people eat less when they are stressed or depressed, but enough people turn to food to have made obesity a society-wide problem.

In the following pages I outline some of the evidence for how our moods influence our consumption of food and other substances. We will see that stressed and depressed people often forgo physical activity and turn instead to easy sources of food energy—often high in calories from sugar and fat. At a time when exercise is an especially valuable ingredient of a healthy lifestyle, we may be just too tired to try. Our moods lie at the center of these relationships, and in the next chapters we will look at how all these relationships play out—and what this means for our health.

CHAPTER 3

How Are Exercise and Mood Related?

LTHOUGH EXERCISE HAS BECOME the Holy Grail, with study after study demonstrating its benefits and the media regularly trumpeting these marvelous results, the patterns of exercise among Americans still do not reflect these realities. Why is this? The answer, in a word, is mood. Negative mood does not put us in the frame of mind to exercise. Even knowing that exercise will alleviate our mood may not be enough of an incentive when we feel drained.

How much more exercise should we be getting? Numerous studies show that people who exercise live longer, have healthier bodies, and are in a more positive psychological state than those who don't.[1] Of course, a possible problem with this kind of evidence is that if we compare people who exercise with those who don't, we can't be certain that the type of people who exercise are not also different in other important respects. For example, it may well be true that a common set of genes influences both a tendency to exercise and the tendency to have better health.[2] Nonetheless, the pattern of evidence does suggest a cause-and-effect relationship between exercise and health, and most scientists believe that such a relationship exists.

But how much exercise do we actually need? From some intriguing anthropological studies carried out by exercise science professor Loren Cordain and his colleagues at Colorado State University, we get an idea of how much exercise our Stone Age ancestors got compared to us.[3] These studies are meaningful because they provide evidence of how much exercise occurred in the lifestyles of the ancestors who provided the genetic blueprints that we live with today.

Those ancestors who survived the travails of a hostile environment with lots of limitations are the ones who passed on their genes. Our bodies are like theirs, and they have bequeathed to us optimal characteristics for survival under the most adverse circumstances. If we wish to know what is best for us, maybe the adaptive lifestyles of these ancestors can give us the answers.

From remains discovered around the world, Cordain and his colleagues concluded that Paleolithic man expended much more energy in physical activity than modern humans do. We would have to carry a twenty-five-pound pack and run 10 miles a day to approximate it. If we were to copy their lifestyle, even thirty minutes of aerobics five days a week—a sizable workout for most—would not measure up. The bodies of these ancestors—as are ours—were specifically adapted for that level of activity, and Cordain and his associates offer evidence that they did not suffer many of the ills common to modern-day humans. At any rate, this evidence, together with many other studies of modern-day people, persuades me that we need much more exercise than we regularly get.[4]

Coming back to exercise in the context of overweight, you can see how essential physical activity really is. At the most basic biological level, over-weight occurs when there is more energy-intensive food ingested than there is energy expenditure through physical activity. In other words, when you eat more than you exercise, you gain weight, and when you exercise more than you eat, you lose weight. It's a simple formula: energy-in must equal energy-out to maintain the same weight.

Of course, other variables must be considered as well. Take, for example, one classic study that searched out pairs of similar-weight individuals who ate vastly different amounts of food.[5] One member of each pair would ingest almost twice as many calories per day as the other, and yet the weight of both remained the same. The reason could not be discovered by careful measures of metabolism at rest or in a variety of activities; there were no apparent constitutional differences in energy requirements. Nor were the differences likely to be due to variations in absorption, as assessed by analyses of elimination products. The large and small eaters did differ in one important respect, however. The large eaters generally walked faster than the small eaters. It appears that in order to maintain the same weight while eating twice as much, one needs to keep up a rapid natural pace of physical activity.

When we see obese people walking slowly, we may assume that the slow speed is due to the extra weight they are carrying. But this research suggests that there may be a difference in tendency toward energetic activity—probably reflected in the way extra food is metabolized—and that this difference causes some people to walk and move faster than others. As you can see, cause and effect is a complicated matter.

A recent *Science* article provided insight into the same problem. Research subjects whose food intake, activity level, and metabolism were observed over eight weeks ate an extra 1,000 calories per day, but the weight gain varied a lot among the participants.[6] For example, one person gained 16 pounds, but another gained only 2. The researchers hypothesized that the differences in weight gain were due to variations in fidgeting, spontaneous muscle contractions, posture, and other related expenditures of energy. This conclusion is intriguing because we all sense that every morsel of food we eat doesn't inevitably add pounds on the scale.[7]

The basic point is still that the same weight can be maintained only when energy-out equals energy-in. How energy is expended is indeed more complicated than at first appears, but it is probably evident to most of us that daily exercise can be an important part of this equation. Large muscle activity expends a proportionately large amount of the energy that we use, as exercise physiologists are well aware. Thus, if we walk an extra 5 miles a day, or even if we just walk faster wherever we go, climb stairs regularly, and so on, we expend more of the energy than comes from the food we eat. If you eat the same amount of food but you engage in more physical activity, you will lose weight—guaranteed.

Exercise and Eating

We know that exercising more while eating the same amount will reduce weight. But if you exercise more, doesn't your appetite increase and make you end up eating more, thus counteracting the reduced energy intake? This could be discouraging to would-be reducers, and even an excuse for not beginning an exercise program—except that it appears not to be true. As counterintuitive as it sounds, the conclusion that more exercise doesn't lead to greater hunger was arrived at by two respected British researchers, John Blundell and Neal King.[8]

Marshaling evidence from many studies of exercise and food intake,

these researchers insist that in the short term there is only a loose coupling between exercise and food intake. In study after study in which
experimental subjects exercised in differing amounts or were sedentary,
food intake was found to change very little.[9] In fact, in a number of studies it was observed that short bouts of exercise actually decreased appetite
(In Chapter 5, I discuss these studies more fully and show how exercising
can help us reduce temporary urges to eat and can be a very important aid
to managing food intake.)

Blundell and King conclude that any association between exercise and
food intake seems to occur only with more intense exercise and over
time. Thus, if your exercise level increases radically and stays at that level,
you will begin to eat more. They argue that in the short term, your
appetite is more related to conditioning, such as is produced by environmental and food cues, as well as other social and cultural influences. What
this means, for example, is that seeing a display of candy bars or knowing
it is time to eat whets our appetite.

We have known for a long time, from classic and well-controlled studies of animals that we now think apply to humans as well that you can
increase exercise a certain amount without increasing appetite. Moderate
exercise first decreases food intake, and appetite increases only when
energy expenditure is much greater.[10] One important implication is that
if you become less active again, your eating habits may continue as before
because they are driven by psychological factors, not physiological need. I
believe that this is one reason people gain weight with age. Energy
declines as a natural function of age, making us less and less active, but we
tend to eat as much as before.

Why Aren't We Exercising More?

Not only are relatively few adults exercising regularly, but there is some
evidence that adults actually may be exercising less today than a decade
ago.[11] The extensive evidence about the value of exercise should have the
gyms packed, the running tracks crowded, and the sidewalks filled with
throngs of people walking. But they aren't. Why not?

The reason many people give for not exercising more is that they are
just too busy. Exercise takes time, and they feel they can't devote the hour
or so a day it requires to stay fit. There is a certain truth to the lack-of-
time argument. People are working more hours and sleeping fewer.[12] And

too little sleep causes negative moods because it leaves us with less energy to keep up with our responsibilities. The inevitable result is increased tension—"tense tiredness," I call it. As we self-regulate with food to change our negative moods, we need more exercise or we will gain weight—and thus the cycle traps us: stress and lack of sleep produce bad moods, which make it difficult to exercise and which induce us to eat more.

Moderate Depression

Stress, lack of sleep, and negative moods contribute to overeating, but could negative moods also be the cause of not exercising? I think so. Although we know we need more exercise to avoid the dreaded overweight, our mood actually stops us from exercising. Negative moods usually involve low energy, or too much tension for the energy available. When your energy is low, you are too tired to exercise. It doesn't matter that exercise will relieve your tiredness and ultimately give you more energy. You just don't feel up to it.

Mary, the thirty-five-year-old woman we met in Chapter 2, knows she should exercise regularly. She has a membership to a health club and plans to share baby-sitting with a neighbor so she can work out three times a week. She followed the plan—for about a week. Then her depression deepened, and her regimen gradually fell by the wayside. She needed energy even more as her feelings of depression increased, but for her the easiest way of getting it was from food.[13]

A key element of Mary's depression was the absence of energy.[14] Everyday activities, especially things she didn't have to do, became just too hard to negotiate. This change in motivation that is governed by reduced energy often is a subtle matter, and it takes a good observer to be aware that a kind of depression is involved. At first it may only be the least necessary obligations that go—things that are on your to-do list, so to speak, but you don't quite get to them. If you find yourself letting things go even though there really is time to do them, moderate depression may be the problem.

One of the things that fell by the wayside for Mary was regular exercise. She knew that it was important, and she fully intended to do it, but her reduced energy made it just too hard to try. She came up with a dozen rationalizations for skipping the exercise, but the real reason was her depression. This is especially ironic because exercise is an excellent aid in managing depression.[15] Mary's continuing low energy and fatigue drove her to find some relief, and energy-intensive food was the solution. As it is for many people, eating proved the easiest way of feeling better.

Some years ago, one of my graduate students and I carried out a study of moderately depressed women in which they carefully rated their depressed times on several occasions, and then on a random schedule they either took a brisk walk or did some sedentary activity.[16] After each walk or sedentary activity, they rated their moods a second time. Unfortunately, most of them dropped out after the first trial or two, even though the exercise reduced their depression. What was the reason? The answer was expressed well by one of my students who said, "When you are depressed, you are just too tired to exercise." Most depressed people thinking about getting themselves out to exercise probably will verify her opinion. One of the best indications of possible depression is tiredness and lack of energy for no apparent reason.[17]

Compare the case of Mary who ate to feel better with that of Stephen, a physician friend of mine in his middle fifties who weighs the same as he did in high school. He has a washboard stomach and a small proportion of body fat. Stephen jogs 2 miles a day, five days a week. But that isn't all the regular exercise he gets. Three days a week he works out with weights, and on top of that he plays tennis several times a week. In addition to being just the right weight, Stephen always seems to be in a positive mood. He rarely eats to self-regulate. He just may be one of those lucky people with the right genes, but I think that his commitment to exercise is crucial. If he misses a day, he feels bad.

Mary, who self-regulates her mood with food, is depressed and unhappy much of the time. She is overweight, and as she looks ahead to her future life, she sees only more of the same. Stephen hardly ever feels depressed. He is very healthy and fit, and not at all overweight. He has arranged the priorities in his life to give him time to exercise an hour or two every single day. Without a doubt, he has had to give up other things to make time for the exercise. But he feels the rewards it brings him far outweigh the sacrifice.

Exercise and Mood: A Vital Connection

In Chapter 1, I said that in our research on ways that people self-regulate, we found exercise to be the single best way of changing a bad mood.

There are at least two good reasons why exercise is such a good mood regulator, and these have to do with the way it changes energy and tension levels, the underlying bases of everyday moods.

It may seem confusing that exercise elevates energy levels. Doesn't exercise use up energy? Don't we know from common sense that exercise tires you out? When a tired (or depressed) person thinks about exercise, it often seems unappealing because it is just too much work. But the fact of the matter is that a moderate amount of exercise usually energizes you.[18]

Try this experiment the next time you are sitting around and feeling tired, especially if you have been sitting for an hour or so. An evening when you are watching TV and feeling hungry for a snack would be an excellent time for it. Rate your energy on a seven-point scale, with 7 being the most energy that you usually feel and 1 being the least. Now get up from the couch and go out for a brisk walk. It may be tough to do because you feel tired, but do it anyway just to see what will happen. Walk at about the speed you would if you were late for an appointment, but without the anxiety you might feel if you really were late. Breathe rhythmically and fairly deeply. Also try to remain fairly erect, but relax the muscles of your body that you do not need for walking or for swinging your arms naturally. Time yourself so that you are gone for just ten minutes.

Something interesting will happen. Within a minute or so you will notice that you aren't as tired as you where when you left the house. Your energy will increase. Keep walking. At the end of ten minutes, rate your energy again on a scale of 1 to 7. You will find that you feel more energetic. Maybe your energy has gone from a 2 to a 3, or maybe from a 2 to a 5. The mere act of exercising for a few short minutes has raised your energy. Your urge for that snack has probably diminished or vanished, too. Make a careful note about your reactions to exercise from this simple experiment if you wish to manage your moods—and your eating—effectively.

In a systematic study that we conducted several years ago, we measured the subjective energy and tension effects of 10 minutes of brisk walking, 30, 60, and 120 minutes after the exercise. What we found was surprising. After only 10 minutes of walking, energy was significantly increased for 60 minutes! We even found a weak but still significant effect

120 minutes after the walk.[19] Think of it: only 10 minutes of brisk walking caused an hour or two of increased energy.[20]

Carefully controlled scientific studies that demonstrate the relationship between exercise and increased energy have been carried out many times now. Take, for example, an extensive naturalistic study done by Lise Gauvin at Concordia University in Canada and Jack Rejeski at Wake Forest University.[21] These exercise scientists studied ninety-three well-educated women of normal height and weight who were enrolled for eleven weeks in fitness classes at the local YMCA. On average, these women were in their early thirties.

Over the eleven-week period these women regularly engaged in bouts of physical activity that lasted twenty minutes or longer: a fitness class, a leisurely or brisk walk, or yoga. The women completed a self-rating of their feelings, both before and after the activity. This naturalistic study eliminated many of the problems that arise in artificial laboratory studies of exercise, because the women were exercising in their natural environments.

The biggest change in mood as a result of these simple bouts of physical activity concerned what the researchers called revitalization: feelings of energy, refreshment, and revival. A mere twenty minutes of physical activity significantly increased the energy of these women and made them feel revitalized. The second biggest mood change concerned what the researchers called positive affect, meaning feeling happy, pleased, and joyful. These feelings also are associated with increased energy and reduced tension. The next biggest mood change occurred in feelings of tranquility such as calmness, peacefulness, and relaxation—in other words, the opposite of tension.

This research is an especially good indication of how a simple physical activity can influence tense tiredness—the basis of bad moods and often the stimulus for overeating. A small amount of physical activity significantly shifted these women's unpleasant tense tired feelings into more positive feelings. The next time you want to feel revitalized, think of this research and try twenty minutes of physical activity. Rate your moods before and after the exercise, and you may be pleasantly surprised by the results.

Exercise and Energy

One late February afternoon a friend and I decided to climb a small mountain at a state park in San Diego near where I live. We started at sea level, where it was cold, but as we continued we started to shed layers—first our jackets, then our outer shirts, leaving us with light T-shirts. By 300 feet we were sweating, even in the chilly air. The heat from the natural generation of energy that our bodies produced was very evident.

If we could have looked inside, we would have seen a host of physiological changes occurring as we hiked up the mountain. When we began, our metabolism increased as glucose was efficiently broken down and energy released in a chemical form called ATP (adenosine triphosphate). In turn, the "energy stations" known as mitochondria in our muscles and elsewhere were activated. Changes were occurring not just at the cellular level, but also throughout many complex systems of our bodies. As we climbed, our heart rate and blood pressure increased. Respiration increased as well, resulting in more oxygen circulating throughout our bodies. Various hormones, such as cortisol and adrenaline, were released into the bloodstream in small amounts, and in certain parts of our brains neurotransmitters and neuromodulators (such as norepinephrine and serotonin) increased in concentration. The energy that was generated came from a pattern of arousal throughout our body.[22] The energetic feeling my friend and I experienced increased *together with* these changes in general bodily arousal.

Energy feelings can be viewed as the uppermost layer in a complex psychophysiological system. As this kind of general bodily arousal increases, feelings of energy increase as well. Although there may be certain physiological changes that are most responsible for increased feelings of energy, no one knows for sure what they are. At the present state of our scientific knowledge, the increased energy feelings appear to be part of a complex pattern of general bodily arousal.[23] I think of energy feelings as the subjective part and increases in metabolism, heart rate, and blood sugar level as the physiological responses that accompany our feelings of energy.

Exercise Intensity and Mood

Remember the experiment I described earlier in which subjects walked briskly for ten minutes and their feelings of energy increased for up to two hours. In that study we also found that the participants experienced decreased feelings of tension. This tension reduction was not as great as the increase in energy, however. With moderate levels of exercise, tension reduction often occurs only as a secondary mood effect. Some other studies also have found that moderate exercise reduces tension sometimes but not always.[24] What about more than moderate exercise? Intense and extended exercise does not increase energy, at least not right afterwards. It uses up your energy and leaves you feeling exhausted. Think about a man who never exercises but who has to run a mile, for example. How would he feel after the run? Depleted of energy. But any tension or anxiety he might have felt before running will have been reduced. The primary mood effect of moderate exercise is increased energy, and the primary mood effect of intense exercise is reduced tension.

A good example was demonstrated in an experiment carried out by exercise scientist Nicolaas Pronk and his associates at Texas A&M University. Twenty-two female volunteers whose average age was forty-five walked, on a motor-driven treadmill, at 3 miles per hour while the grade was gradually raised—about 2.5 percent every three minutes.[25] As you can imagine, this is a demanding form of exercise, and before long each participant indicated that she could no longer continue. On average, this took about twenty-two minutes.

The researchers asked each participant to rate her mood before she began on the treadmill and immediately after stopping. As you might expect, some of the biggest mood changes that the researchers found were decreased feelings of vigor and energy, and increased feelings of fatigue. But tension and anxiety also decreased significantly. These subjects had engaged in heavy exercise—just as you might if you worked out really hard at a gym—and they felt exhausted, but their tension had decreased significantly.

This tension reduction is exactly what many of my students have described experiencing after their intense workouts, and indeed I have experienced it myself, but not all studies support it. For example, in a widely cited study, British scientist Andrew Steptoe found that moderate exercise increased energy and that intense exercise actually increased tension.[26]

Part of the reason for this discrepancy may be found in research conducted by John Raglin and his associates at Indiana University, which suggests that engaging in heavy exercise may increase your anxiety temporarily, but then it decreases after a few minutes and remains low.[27] In one experiment that showed this, subjects peddled an exercise bicycle for twenty minutes at 70 percent VO_2 peak.[28] VO_2 peak can be thought of as something like maximum heart rate, and this twenty-minute task was certainly a heavy workload. Light and moderate workloads of 40 percent and 60 percent VO_2 peak also were used in two other conditions.

When these researchers analyzed systematic self-ratings from the subjects of their anxiety levels, they found that, at the highest workload, anxiety was significantly increased five minutes after finishing, but by one hour it was significantly decreased. And it remained low at two hours when the last ratings were taken. In the light and moderate workloads (40 percent and 60 percent VO_2 peak), anxiety was significantly lowered at five minutes after exercise, and it remained low for the remaining two hours. From this, it appears that heavy exercise may increase tension for a short while right after the workout, but in a few minutes the anxiety is gone and it remains low for some time.[29]

These various studies provide a lot of good information for self-management of mood. If you are feeling a bit low and could use a burst of energy, a short, brisk walk will probably do the trick. But suppose you have had a very stressful day and you are feeling tense and wound up. This may call for a trip to the gym and a heavy workout. But don't be alarmed if, in the course of the workout, your tension increases slightly as you exercise. The final result is likely to be calmness that will last for hours. The calmness is good, but what about the energy decline that occurs with a heavy workout? I have found that after an hour or two of recovery from a heavy workout, often there is a burst of energy that lasts for quite a while.

Not long ago, one of my former students, Paula, told me of just such an energy charge. After work she was wound up with the tension that came from an overwhelming schedule of meetings and demands. She felt ready to burst as she headed for the gym and a hard aerobics class. Before the class she loosened up and worked with weights a bit, then she hit the aerobics floor. An hour later she was exhausted as she headed home, but it was too early for bed. After a light supper and some amusing TV, she started to feel energized, and the reports she had brought home with her caught her attention. Although she was dreading this extra work, she now plunged into it with vigor, working well into the evening. She wasn't surprised about the energy surge. She was anticipating it from experience. Paula knows how to manage her moods very well.

Weight Training and Mood

Weight training is becoming popular nowadays, and it is often recommended as a way of increasing metabolically active muscle mass that is beneficial in weight loss. Resistance training such as the moderate-intensity lifting that Paula used in conjunction with her aerobics class has become common. But unlike the effects of aerobic exercise, little research has focused on weight training and mood.

In one review of a few early studies, no anxiety reduction was found.[30] But in another more recent study that took careful measures of anxiety for an hour after weight lifting, exercise scientist John Raglin required college athletes to engage for thirty minutes in various kinds of weight training, and each person lifted at 70 percent to 80 percent of his or her one-repetition maximum—a fairly intensive task.[31] These students' self-rated anxiety increased significantly immediately after lifting but returned to baseline levels twenty minutes after the exercise and fell below baseline 60 minutes after it. The anxiety reduction Raglin found was not statistically significant, but exercise scientist Patrick O'Connor and his associates did find that resistance exercise significantly reduced anxiety sixty minutes after the exercise. They also established that moderately intensive exercise (60 percent VO_2 max) reduced anxiety the most.[32]

Interpreting these various results is difficult because there is too little research to make any claims, but it appears that heavy lifting may temporarily increase tension and anxiety, then relieve them. After an hour or so feelings of anxiety are reduced. I know of no research on how weight lifting affects energy, which we will need to know in order to understand the overall mood effects. Even if tension is increased, if energy is increased as well, the effect could be quite positive. The other shortcoming in the research that has been done is that we don't know enough about how different intensities of weight lifting affect people's mood.

I believe that muscle tension contributes a great deal to negative moods. For example, when you are in a bad mood you often have a tight neck, shoulders, and back. Therefore, it makes sense that moderate lifting ultimately relaxes your muscles and leaves you in a much better mood. At different times, try weight training at various intensities and pay attention to your energy and tension levels immediately afterward and for the next hour or two. Your self-observations can be of great value to you in learning to manage your mood.

Too Much Exercise

For most Americans, increasing the level of physical activity will yield only positive effects. But as a general biological principle it must be said that there is some intensity and degree of exercise that will not be beneficial. When Hans Selye, the famous Canadian endocrinologist, conducted many of his early pioneering studies of stress, he used forced exercise with animals as a way of stressing them. [33] Even though exercise is often prescribed as a form of stress management today, it is clear that too much exercise can be detrimental.

An example of excessive exercise comes from the overtraining of athletes, which can result not only in various physical disabilities but in pervasive fatigue and mood disorders. In one recent study of long-distance runners, the athletes' mood state was the best indication of whether or not they had exercised excessively. [34] We also see examples of excessive exercise and a resultant negative mood state with eating disorders, especially anorexia nervosa. [35] In one British study of twenty-one anorexic women, for example, the researchers concluded that the women showed a negative addiction to exercise. [36] They continued to exercise when they were sick or injured, and they experienced mood symptoms of withdrawal if their exercise was prevented. The experience of these anorexics illustrates the powerful effect that exercise has on mood.

The Pleasure of Exercise

Although it may be hard to begin an exercise program, and although intense exercise can exhaust you, once it is done (and not overdone), the ultimate effect is usually pleasure. If you doubt this, ask anyone who exercises regularly. He may give you lots of reasons for exercising, but he will also tell you that it makes him feel good. It elevates his mood.

The fact that physical activity creates feelings of pleasure makes sense when you realize that energy increases with exercise, especially moderate exercise. Energy feels good, and exercise is one of the most reliable producers of this pleasurable feeling. Exercise is also pleasurable because it reduces tension and anxiety. Other mood-related states are also influenced by exercise, but I believe that energy and feelings of tension are central to all of them.

The pleasure of exercise is also evident in studies of how people evaluate themselves. Although not unequivocal, a sizable body of scientific research suggests that exercise raises self-esteem.[37] This is a complicated research area. For example, self-esteem is frequently measured as a trait that is relatively unchanging, and thus some researchers don't think it can be affected by the short-term changes that occur from a single bout of exercise. They assume that increased physical conditioning through exercise leaves you feeling better about yourself overall, but that at any one time it has little effect on self-esteem. I believe, however, that your level of self-esteem changes continuously and may be affected by even a small amount of exercise.

In a study of college students that Joan Rubadeau and I conducted some years ago, we found that self-esteem varied considerably on different days. College students gave us self-ratings of self-esteem as well as energy and tension ratings many times over several weeks. One clear-cut finding was that energy level significantly predicted self-esteem.[38] In other words, at any given time the more energetic a student felt, the higher she rated her self-esteem. From the majority of studies that have been done on exercise and self-esteem, it appears that people rate themselves more positively when they exercise.[39]

Related to self-esteem is something called self-efficacy, or the belief that you can be successful at any particular task. Self-efficacy has received a lot of attention by psychotherapists because it is thought to be the most important part of behavior change.[40] In other words, your belief that you can accomplish something is the best predictor of your success at that task. Exercise strengthens self-efficacy, especially in relation to physical capabilities.[41] Psychological well-being is still another characteristic that is strengthened by exercise.[42]

Other mood changes from exercise have the effect of increased pleasure as well. For example, I have already discussed how exercise decreases moderate depression, at least temporarily. And since depression is a condition of reduced energy and heightened tension, exercise may well bring about its effect by changing these feelings. Anyone doubting the pleasurable effect of even a temporary decrease in depression should realize that depression is a very unpleasant state. For example, in one study of people who had experienced both depression and severe physical pain, these unfortunate individuals indicated that, if given the choice, they would rather have the pain.[43] Clearly, relief from feelings of depression is pleasurable.

It must be said, of course, that the depression-reducing effects of exercise aren't always obvious. You will recall the depressed women who gave up the walking that was reducing their depression because they were too tired to do it. It is sometimes necessary to make the cognitive connection between exercise and elevated mood in order to motivate yourself to begin exercising.

Still another way that exercise yields pleasure, but that most people do not think about, has to do with stress management. If we can control the negative effects of stress, we will feel pleasure. A sizable scientific literature shows that exercise seems to inoculate us against stress.[44] A good example of how exercise seems to bolster people against stress comes from a study recently conducted by British psychologist Andrew Steptoe and his colleagues.[45] They observed the stress experiences of seventy-three men and women over twelve days by asking them to fill in a diary at the end of each day, in which they rated daily stress experiences that are quite common (for example, "I had too many things to do"). The subjects of this study exercised sometimes but not every day, so it was possible to study their reactions to stress on days when they exercised compared to days when they didn't. The results, which were analyzed by type of person, were enlightening. Less anxious people reported fewer stressful events on the days when they exercised. Other people reported that potentially stressful events were nonstressful on days when they exercised. In an interesting additional finding, mood ratings seemed to indicate that the positive mood changes produced by the exercise were more important than the reduced tension. Once again, this suggests that energy enhancement is a critical part of the enjoyment of exercise.

Given the pleasure that exercise can produce, we must once again question why most people are exercise-starved.

Negative Moods: A Double-Edged Sword

At the beginning of this chapter, I said that people are exercising less than they should and that moods often are the cause. But there is a paradox here: moods both stop us from exercising and can encourage or stimulate our exercise. Consider how this works.

Our moods often inhibit our exercise moment by moment, and ultimately day by day, because they lie at the base of a lack of resolve to get up and move. When a good time for exercise arises, we think about getting started. If we lack energy—for example, if we are feeling slightly depressed—this mood leads us to consider the anticipated exercise in a negative way. It's a kind of unconscious mental process that occurs so rapidly that it usually escapes our awareness.

To see more clearly the paradox I am speaking about, compare the way that our moods inhibit us from exercising with some findings from a recent study that one of my students and I conducted.[46] Evana Hsiao and I designed a survey to learn more about why people exercise. If you regularly go to a gym or health club you will see the same people over and over. It must take them lots of time to do this, and by watching their huffing and puffing you can see that the exercise takes lots of effort. What motivates them?

Our study grew out of my theory that if exercise is such a good mood regulator and if it feels good to decrease negative moods and elevate positive moods, people should be motivated to continue exercising. This follows from well-known principles of positive reinforcement but stands in stark contrast to the epidemic of inactivity. We reasoned that the mood elevation that comes from exercise is subtle but the motivation to avoid exercising because of tiredness can be very powerful. It may take time and experience to recognize how exercise elevates mood. In other words, as people have more experience with exercise, they should begin to use this kind of physical activity to regulate their moods.

To test these ideas, we systematically questioned a representative group of people who had just joined a health club and compared their reasons for exercise with the reasons given by those who had exercised for a year or more. We found that the more experience people had with exercising, the more they gave mood regulation as a reason to do it. Health club members often began exercising to improve their physical appearance, but after a year or more that motivation had decreased. Mood became significantly more important as a reason. I don't know whether the regular exercisers actually think about the way the exercise will make them feel each time they begin, but they do become more aware of this motivation as they exercise more. Thus it is easier to get up and do it, knowing they will feel better later.

Let's consider how developing an exercise program might work in practical terms. For you to be motivated to begin and, more important, to continue an exercise program, first, you must make it a high priority. Time must be allotted for it, even when it interferes with other parts of your life. Giving exercise a high priority can come from an understanding of how regular physical activity is essential for health and happiness.

Next, it is important that exercise be pleasurable.[47] Most forms of exercise fulfill this requirement, but I am a believer in moderate exercise—the kind that feels good each time you do it. As I observe exercisers working out, especially beginners, I notice that they often are doing too much. It's true that you can get into moderately good physical condition in mere weeks by pressing yourself hard, but a pressing exercise schedule may not be fun. The pleasure of exercise is what will keep you motivated, and the more immediate and continuous the pleasure is, the more you will stick with it.

Continuing to exercise is the problem for most people. If it is to be a lifelong practice, exercise must become an integral part of your lifestyle. Your motivation to continue will increase if you can avoid the impatience that pushes you to get into good physical shape quickly, at the cost of immediate pleasure. A moderate exercise schedule in which you gradually push yourself to do more may take three times as long to put you into shape, but good conditioning will occur and, more important, the motivation to continue will remain high. The rule should be to make exercise fun and pleasurable each time it occurs.

Finally, there is the problem of exercising when at that moment you feel too tired or depressed to do it. To overcome this pitfall you must become aware of how good you will feel after you exercise and resolve to continue no matter how unpleasant it appears. You can use simple tricks to fool yourself. For example, don't think about walking for a half-hour at a rapid pace. Just set out to walk slowly to the corner. This slow walk often will increase your energy, and when you get to the corner you will feel like walking another block, and so on. Your body will help you make that decision by yielding more energy; this is the way moods and thoughts interact.[48]

Exercise, Nutrition, and Weight Control

James Rippe, the well-known medical researcher from Tufts University, and his associate, Stacey Hess, recently reviewed the literature on weight loss and concluded that a combination of increased physical activity and sound nutrition is the most effective approach to losing weight—and keeping it off.[49] I believe that a very important reason for this effectiveness has to do with the way exercise influences mood and, in turn, the effect of mood on unnecessary eating. Putting two bodies of evidence together—how exercise affects mood and how mood affects eating—leads to convincing conclusions.

Before considering mood as a primary explanation for effective maintenance of weight loss, let us consider some other possibilities. Although there is a consensus among researchers that eating less is not as effective for weight loss by itself as it is when combined with exercise,[50] comparisons between exercise and eating less show that restricting your diet has the quickest effect. Think about it. To burn 600 calories you would have to exercise intensely for an hour, but in a couple of minutes, with no trouble at all, you could take in over twice that number of calories by eating a Big Mac, french fries, and a soda.[51] Exercise alone doesn't do the trick—at least at the level of physical activity that most people are likely to do.

Nevertheless, there could be a number of reasons why exercise combined with eating less is so effective, in addition to the obvious fact of greater calorie reduction when the two occur together. For example, exercise raises your resting metabolic rate, so even when you are not exercising you are burning more calories. Furthermore, losing weight tends to reduce resting metabolic rate, and exercise can at least partially counteract this effect. (But the effects of raising or maintaining resting metabolic rate may have been overemphasized. When considering the actual effect, it's not that great.)[52]

Another reason for the success of combined exercise and calorie restriction is that exercise allows you to maintain lean muscle mass that otherwise would be reduced if you only restricted your diet. This could be important because muscle tissue is much more active metabolically than fat, and therefore losing muscle tissue lowers resting metabolic rate. Once again, although this can be an important reason for exercising while losing weight, it probably isn't significant enough to account for the observed differences in success of weight loss when exercise is employed.

Now let's come back to mood. I believe that an often overlooked reason for the success of physical activity together with calorie restriction is that exercise elevates your mood, and your mood has an important effect on what and how much you eat. In the previous pages, I described study after study showing the positive effects of exercise on mood, and in the next chapter I will carefully consider research that shows how negative moods create food urges and appetites for food that you do not need. People who exercise and restrict calorie intake feel better and do not rely on food as much to improve their moods. I believe that the basis of this exercise effect is the increased energy and reduced tension that it produces. Food gives pleasure; it makes you feel better. So when you are feeling unhappy, depressed, or otherwise low, you know that a snack will raise your spirits. But if your spirits can be raised by exercise, you do not need the extra food.

Another reason why people who exercise and eat less are more successful at maintaining their weight loss has to do with self-esteem, and, of course, this is related to mood as well. When you exercise you feel good about yourself, and it is easier to withstand the temptation of food. Tension and low energy occur in every person's life from time to time, and it is then that the forbidden foods are most attractive. But resisting that attraction often is easier when you know you are doing something positive for yourself—a regular exercise program, for example—and this gives you the strength to avoid overeating.

Not only are negative moods in general improved by exercise, but exercise helps us overcome specific moods, such as mild depression. Depression can be a potent stimulus for overeating. Finally, it is likely that reactions to stress are reduced by exercise. Stress often leads us to overeat or to eat the wrong kinds of food. In all these ways, combining exercise with eating less is likely to be an effective strategy for maintaining weight loss, but it is important to realize that the effectiveness is closely related to maintaining a positive mood.

The evidence about how moods influence the way we eat is broad and solid. It is often summarized under the term "emotional eating," and in the next chapter I will examine this topic in detail.

CHAPTER 4

Emotional Eating

A T MY LAST VISIT to the local bookstore, I counted 132 books on diet, 35 books on food-counters, and 110 books on general nutrition—all recently published and currently in print. In addition, over 450 special diet cookbooks tell readers how to prepare low-calorie and low-fat meals and how to choose foods especially important for weight control.

Most of these books have a bottom line: how to make yourself thin. They focus on which foods to eat and not to eat, particular combinations of foods that purport to melt pounds away and enhance well-being. Diets are offered that will not only cure illness but strengthen self-esteem, along with controlling weight, of course. Consider, for example, the following quotes taken from several widely selling books:

- You'll enhance your brain's mood chemistry to deliver the self-esteem, mental energy, vigor and power to hold the line against foods that make you fat instead of depending on stubborn willpower to endure hunger.
- Fight disease the easy way—discover how veggies, fruits, and grains can help save your life.
- [These dietary supplements will allow you to] improve your memory and concentration. Increase your mental endurance. Temper and prevent depression.
- For many of us, mood and energy problems are a result of what we

49

eat and how we live. In most cases, making a few simple choices in what and when we eat could be all it takes to feel better.

- This Zone state of exceptional health is well-known to champion athletes. Your own journey toward it can begin with your next meal. You will no longer think of food as merely an item of pleasure or a means to appease hunger. Food is your medicine and your ticket to that state of ultimate body balance, strength and great health in the Zone.[1]

A moment's consideration of these claims must leave the intelligent reader with some question about their truth, if not outright disbelief. If easy dieting is so beneficial, why are so many people still on diets? At any one time, over a third of the population is dieting—that's tens of millions of people.[2] But we are not getting thinner. Is it because people haven't yet read these books and grasped their wisdom? Is it just a matter of getting the information out to the public? Or is it possible that there is some exaggeration in many of these popular books, that the scientific evidence isn't as clear as the reader is led to believe, that in everyday life losing weight isn't quite so easy?

Given all the hype, when a diet claim is provided the first question that should spring to mind is, How does the writer know this? When science is given as proof of food claims, the savvy reader must try to understand the general nature of the studies that were done and just what they showed. These studies are not usually so technical that the procedures, as well as the findings, can't be understood by nonscientists.[3]

Thinking about the scientific evidence behind books that claim the imprimatur of science, I am reminded of some research done by Christina Pechan, one of my best advanced psychology students. She analyzed the scientific basis of a best-selling book that promises great benefits from a diet emphasizing the value of certain percentages of proteins, carbohydrates, and fats. This book assures the reader that there is solid scientific evidence to support these claims. But the references offered at the back of the book do not prove its central claims. The author draws conclusions that go beyond the available scientific evidence. This is not to say that the diet has no value, but only that it has not been scientifically proven.

Is it possible that books with no established scientific basis still may offer a valuable diet? Possibly. The published science tends to lag behind actual food practices that many people may be trying and finding successful.[4]

Do Special Diets Produce Lasting Weight Loss?

Most of the popular diet books focus on particular food combinations as keys to weight loss.[5] It is easy to see why: controlling your moods is much harder than following a certain diet. Unfortunately, the question of whether particular foods, especially unusual food combinations, can produce lasting weight loss remains unanswered.

In his recent book, *Eat, Drink, and Be Merry*, media physician Dean Edell reviews various kinds of fad diets that are on the market.[6] Edell, well known for being up on the latest scientific evidence, argues that the many diets (including the different kinds of high-protein plans) help you to lose weight initially, often through reduced water retention, and this is why they generate such believers. But, he says, the long-term medical consequences, and the inevitable regained weight when you go off the diet, make them poor strategies for weight management. Evaluating a range of nonstandard diets, his conclusion—eat whatever you want, but eat less of it—will undoubtedly work, so long as your activity level remains the same.

In relation to high protein diets and Edell's idea of eating less, I was particularly struck with the fact that although a friend of mine who has been on such a diet is now eating less, largely because she finds less food to her liking, she still wants more food. This isn't the usual explanation for weight loss from such diets, as proponents argue that you can eat as much as you want as long as you eat certain kinds of foods. However, eating less could be the ultimate result of such diets if certain foods are not liked in the proportions allowed. One reason not usually assumed for weight loss with such diets could have to do with their requirement that you scrutinize what you eat to maintain the proper proportions of foods. Such self-monitoring usually results in eating less—for a while. This is the *reactivity effect* documented by behaviorists, but unfortunately it is short-lived and you tend to go back to eating as much as you did before.[7]

In any event, eating less than you want is easier to say than do. It often results in food cravings and persistent hunger that can be temporarily resisted, but eventually, when your resources are low, your resolve finally crumbles and the diet is gone. Getting to the core of food cravings and hunger is the key. Undoubtedly, what you eat is important in weight control, especially with short-term weight loss, but keeping that weight off is another matter. If you eat a lot of energy-intensive food (like junk food) you will gain weight, especially if you don't exercise more to counteract it, but if you eat sensibly, and reduce the portions that you eat, you will lose weight.[8] Once the weight is lost, however, often through some supreme act of willpower, how do you keep it off? How do you maintain the willpower? Unfortunately, the statistics for success are very bad: over 90 percent of people who lose weight gain it back.[9] This is where your moods and emotional eating—that is, eating driven by negative feelings like depression and anxiety—enter the picture. Your moods may be influenced by the food you eat, but even more important, your moods influence your food urges and your motivation to eat or not eat over time, especially your motivation to keep a particular diet as a lifestyle change.

What should you eat to lose weight? *Unusual* food combinations such as those found in high protein diets that are different from well-known dietary standards may result in weight loss, but reliable scientific evidence for lasting change simply doesn't exist. Nutrition experts already know, as do many people in the general population, how to eat properly for optimal weight loss. These principles are not mysterious. What isn't well known is how to keep the weight off once it is lost. Here is where understanding mood makes a real contribution.

How Moods Influence Eating

My theory about eating and exercise is based on a body of research. In one review of more than fifty scientific studies Richard Ganley summarized a wide variety of evidence that much obesity is based on emotional eating.[10] In these studies the emotions or moods that precede overeating invariably were described as depression, anxiety, anger, boredom, and loneliness— negative moods. And I have found that these negative moods usually have in common low energy and increased tension. As people attempt to change or self-regulate these negative states with food they tend to overeat.

Negative moods often occur before we overeat, as numerous studies have shown.[11] A recent episode of the popular television show *Frasier* illustrated the instinctive knowledge we have about this emotional eating. Frasier has lost his job as a radio psychologist, and he tells his family and friends that he's not having a problem with it; being unemployed just gives him more time for his other pursuits, he maintains. But as time passes, he gets fatter and fatter, and as we see him in subsequent scenes he is eating continuously. The writers don't even bother explaining his motivation to overeat. Every viewer knows why it is happening.[12]

Sometimes individual differences play a role in emotional eating. That is, negative emotions that lead to diet breaking may regularly cause overeating for some *types* of people more than for others. We know, for example, that "restrained eaters"—those on some kind of diet—are more likely to show emotional eating than nondieters. Of course, in today's society we may ask, Who isn't on a diet? We will deal more with these individual differences in a later section.

Food Urges and Self-Regulation

Positive moods sometimes cause overeating, as in a celebration or good social company, but usually negative moods are the cause.[13] The food temporarily changes our mood and makes us feel better. In particular, it temporarily raises energy or reduces tension, or both, thus resulting in overall mood improvement. Over many occasions, eating habits develop in just this way so that we are conditioned to turn to food when a negative mood hits. This mood regulation through food is a continual moment-to-moment process that occurs as we respond to our feelings of tension and low energy by eating some energy-generating food. Tension and low energy—the condition I call tense tiredness—often influence us when we think about good-tasting food we might find in our kitchen or in the candy machine at work. Frequently, this leads to an internal dialog in which competing thoughts race through our minds reminding us of the "good" reasons why the forbidden food should be eaten now, countered by guilty thoughts about indulging. As any dieter knows, this battle can be complex and can go on for long periods before it is temporarily resolved by a gritting-of-the-teeth effort and avoidance or, far too often, by succumbing to the temptation.

A few years ago, an excellent study illustrating many of these points was conducted by Andrew Hill and Lisa Heaton-Brown, two British biopsychologists who set out to study the experience of food cravings.[14] Most of us have these cravings when we aren't especially in need of food, and yet there they are—those gnawing feelings that we want something good to eat. In one study of over 1,000 college students, 97 percent of women and 68 percent of men indicated that they experience food cravings, and that at least half the time they indulge them.[15] If we're breaking a diet, this can crumple our resolve and open the floodgates to a bout of unrestrained eating. It has what some researchers call a snowballing effect.[16] But where do these cravings come from and how do they motivate us to overeat? If these questions could be answered, it might be possible to gain some effective control. The English study provides good answers to at least some of these questions.

Unlike many of the past studies that have been done on food craving, which asked people to report on past experiences, this study analyzed the cravings while they were occurring. These researchers enlisted the help of a group of dedicated women who kept track of their food desires over five-week periods. They also rated their moods before and after the cravings, thus allowing us to see what moods preceded the cravings and how eating changed those moods. The research participants ranged from twenty to fifty-seven years of age, and the average woman wasn't overweight.

One interesting finding about the food urges that these women experienced was that chocolate was the desired food almost half the time.[17] The next most common craving was for "something sweet," and savory foods were sometimes the object of the craving. Careful records indicated that four out of five times when the cravings occurred, the women ended up eating something, and 92 percent of the time it was the desired food that was eaten. Usually no longer than fifteen minutes passed between the time the craving began and the time the craved food was eaten.

This is a good description of a common way of overeating. Thoughts and urges for food arise. We start thinking about the food, imagining how good it will taste. Then we begin to crave it. Not long after that, we eat it. Usually the object of our urge is an energy-intensive food, often something loaded with sugar or fat and often something we know we shouldn't eat if our diet is to be kept.

Now let's look at certain results from this study a little more carefully. Sixty percent of the time these women first *thought* about the food and then the craving began. If you are trying to stop food cravings, a valuable tool for control comes from knowing that thoughts about the food often arise before the urges and before the eating. Our thoughts and feelings are closely linked. If we can control one, the other often can be controlled as well. Changing our thoughts often changes our feelings.

In addition to studying thinking patterns, these scientists also focused on feelings or moods that seemed to signal the onset of food cravings. Each time a craving occurred, self-ratings were made, and it was clear that the women commonly felt tense when the urges appeared and much less tense after the urge—usually after eating. With the passing of the urge came a combination of higher energy and reduced tension, an increase in something mood researchers call hedonic tone.[18] Self-rated energy also rose, especially when the urges were for certain foods. Lastly, hunger was reduced. One important thing to notice is that feelings of tension, low energy, and hunger existed together.[19]

This study provides a good picture of how negative moods involving tension and reduced energy appear to activate overeating, and how food seems to lift those moods. We can look at this as an illustration of how a bad food habit is formed. First there is the negative mood. Then we think about a food that will change it. Finally, we succumb to the urge to eat the food. Quickly, we experience the reward and feel better—a positive mood occurs. We know from decades of behavioral research that habits are formed and continued in just this way. In technical terms, scientists talk about a stimulus, a response, and a reinforcement.[20] The next time we feel that negative mood, we know what will change it—at least in the short term.

Why do negative moods, and particularly tension and low energy, lead us to eat? These feelings are uncomfortable, and when uncomfortable feelings occur we naturally try to change them to feel better. Of course, you can just accept the discomfort and live with it, but most people don't have that kind of self-control. They want to feel better right away. Or even if they maintain their self-control for a while, eventually it breaks down. Eating is the easiest way to feel better. It may only be temporary, and it may cause us to feel guilty, but food is easy, it tastes good, and it makes us feel better right away. The immediacy of this feeling is very important to us especially when we reach that point at which we must escape from a negative mood right away. By the way, this condition of urgency is often a prescription for bingeing.

Why does good-tasting food make us feel better? Obviously we enjoy its taste, but the truth is more complicated than that. Good-tasting foods such as simple sugars and fats tend to metabolize rapidly and to raise our blood sugar quickly. Energy is the immediate result. This energy counteracts the tense tiredness that we might be feeling.[21] It is the reinforcement that controls the habit.

Once established, habits tend to drive our behavior and to override our most intense resolve. To use our food illustration, at least some of the time the food must allow us to escape from that negative mood, that very unpleasant tense tired state, or the habit dies out—scientists call that extinction. And the more times we eat as a way of escaping our bad moods, the stronger the habit becomes. What this means for many people is that years of training produce habits that are extremely hard to break— but not impossible.

Of course, much of the time this whole process happens unconsciously, or at a low level of consciousness, as you would expect from years of habit training. It might have begun when we weren't even able to talk and our mothers reacted to our tears by giving us something good to eat. With this kind of conditioning, our thoughts about food become closely linked to negative moods, and particularly to low energy and tension. The thoughts may be the first conscious reactions, but they are part of a learned pattern. Or the habit formation may happen when we are older. At one bad time in our lives we may discover that gorging on good-tasting food made us feel better. A drug could have been one escape route, and many addicts got there in just this way, but most of us are leery of the side effects of drugs. Food is the more likely choice. It is readily available, and it is constantly in our consciousness from media, advertising, and store displays. It is natural to think about food when we need energy and we are feeling tense.

The process by which bad food habits control us is very insidious. These habits sneak up on us and gradually control our consciousness and our eating behavior. If we want to change the outcome of that process, we must understand what is happening.

Triggers to Overeating

Are there triggers to overeating? If so, can we avoid them? An interesting study by three researchers from the University of Kansas focused on so-called triggers.[22] The women studied in this research included a normal-weight group, an overweight group (10 percent above ideal), and an obese group (at least 20 percent above ideal). The women in the latter two groups were considered weight cyclers—they had lost and regained more than ten pounds in the last two years. The research involved intensive hour-long structured interviews that focused on recent episodes of overeating.

All the women experienced the same triggers for overeating, but those with identified food problems reacted more strongly to these prompts. One triggering condition was planned overeating. This occurred when the women overate while celebrating a special occasion. Forty-two percent of the normal-weight women did this, while 100 percent of the overweight women reported this common trigger.

Such planned overeating is a key concept in understanding why we overeat and how this behavior is related to our moods. We often self-regulate our moods not only to escape an unpleasant condition such as tense tiredness, but also to feel very good when our moods are otherwise just all right. A special celebration gives us license to break our dietary prohibitions and to indulge.[23]

These women probably recognized that they were going to gain weight from the unnecessary food, but they probably rationalized it because of a special occasion, and special occasions demand being in a good mood regardless of the dietary consequences. Everyone knows about gaining weight around the holidays. We have lots of parties and special occasions just in order to raise our moods—and society reinforces this behavior around Thanksgiving, Christmas, and New Year's, for example, with plenty of advertising. Retailers count on it. (This is not to mention the overeating needed to self-regulate the negative moods that the holidays cause in some people.)

An interesting difference between the normal-weight participants and the women who were overweight but not obese in this study was that the normal-weight participants overate in the company of friends and family members, but the overweight women overate when they were alone. Overeating while alone may have to do with being especially conscious of the disapproval of others or just with shame. Aside from the times when they engaged in planned overeating, another interesting finding in this research was that all the overweight and obese participants ate either in the afternoon or the evening. As we shall see later, daily energy cycles are likely to influence overeating. In the afternoon, many people experience drops in energy, and as the evening progresses energy reaches the lowest point of the day for most individuals. The resultant tiredness leaves people vulnerable to tension. This tense tiredness is exactly the state that motivates people to eat as a kind of self-regulation.

Another pattern associated with overeating in the Kansas research was what the researchers called power/control. Most, but not all, of the normal-weight subjects had a feeling of personal control before and during the overeating, but the overweight and obese women felt much less control. Again, an out-of-control feeling is common among those who suffer from eating problems, but most people probably experience this feeling to a lesser or greater degree from time to time when they have the urge to overindulge.

The most important findings of the research for our interest concern the way that unpleasant feelings were triggers to overeating. Both the normal-weight participants and the weight cyclers experienced the same negative moods before eating and the same relief from those negative feelings during and after eating. The normal-weight participants, however, showed fewer of these effects than the overweight and obese women. This makes sense when we realize that people with eating problems often act more intensely than normal-weight people with regard to food, even though everyone may have the same general reactions.

Considering all the women in the study, almost a third felt tired, bored, or lonely before overeating. Not surprisingly, eating allayed these feelings. While they ate, only 5 percent of the women had these negative feelings, and after they ate, only 7 percent did. You could say that the low energy that usually characterizes these negative states drove these women to eat, and as proof of that, the negative feelings diminished when they ate.

Anxiety, tension, and stress were other feelings that changed before and after eating. Angry and depressed feelings also were reported, and these feelings were lessened by eating as well. But after the eating episode was over, the women felt about as angry and depressed as they had before, and this is consistent with other research showing that negative feelings, especially guilt, often follow a period of overeating. Nevertheless, it is the actual act of eating that reinforces the habit.[24]

Tiredness and Tension

Another recent study conducted by Finnish researchers focused on reasons people began to eat and stopped eating. The subjects were 114 obese

individuals who kept self-monitoring diaries over twenty-four-hour periods.[25] Their job was to complete self-ratings before and after every eating
episode. Once again, tension and tiredness were the feelings that changed
from the beginning to the end of the eating. Every one of the participants
felt reduced tension after eating, but this effect was most reliable in the
less obese half of the group. And every one felt significantly less tired after
eating—again the energizing effect of food that I spoke about earlier.[26]
One other interesting result was that the most obese participants felt significantly happier after eating, which illustrates the reinforcing effect that
food has on habits to eat. Now let us consider other research in which
dieters are confronted with temptations to break their diets.

Relapse Among Dieters

Every person trying to lose weight is familiar with temptations to eat
unnecessarily and, all too often, with failures. The resolve to diet is often
formulated during a relatively good mood and not after a difficult day
when we are feeling tense and tired. It takes a certain amount of energy to
make a plan and resolve to carry it out.

But what about the inevitable temptations to lapse? These periods
when the diet is broken are crucial to understanding weight gain and loss,
not necessarily because of the additional food that is eaten at that moment
but because the broken resolve shatters your willpower and often leads to
unrestrained eating that can go on for a long time. It is as though we give
up when our willpower is broken. Understanding the causes of these
lapses might go a long way toward eliminating the broken diets.

Carlos Grilo, Saul Shiffman, and Rena Wing studied dieters who were
all overweight and most of whom had long-standing weight problems (on
the average they were 60 percent over normal body weight) and extensive
histories of failed diets. Participants described recent incidents of overeating or being highly tempted to do so.[27]

In the various relapse crises, as the researchers called them, negative
moods or feelings—including tension, anxiety, anger, tiredness, or a
down feeling—were present in the majority of cases in which overeating
occurred (54 percent). It seems apparent that the study participants
were motivated to self-regulate their low energy levels by eating, and
this is why the relapses occurred. The researchers grouped the relapse

crises into three common patterns: mealtimes, low arousal periods (such as being tired), and times when the subjects recognized being emotionally upset. Other people were present during mealtimes, and socializing was the common activity. But, like the study of food triggers described earlier, in this research positive emotions could sometimes also be present when overeating occurred. In the pattern associated with being emotionally upset, anger, depression, or anxiety were commonly present (in 91 percent of the cases). The third pattern these researchers found, which they called low arousal, was a state that many of the subjects described as feeling tired (low energy) or down, for example.[28] A "down" feeling is often a euphemism for moderate depression, and it is usually characterized by a pattern of decreased energy and moderately increased tension.

Many people aren't aware of the importance of this low-energy state as a cause of overeating, but it is often the case. The so-called crises of these dieters all occurred in the afternoon and evening, times when energy begins to decline for most people. The average relapse crisis for these subjects occurred at 4:34 P.M. For most people, energy sinks in the late afternoon, and this is an especially dangerous time for food temptations. In addition, the crises of these dieters usually occurred when they were at least moderately hungry (four hours and ten minutes since the last meal). Thus, hunger and its accompanying low energy and increased tension could be expected to result in a great temptation to eat and, as we can see in this case, in temptations to overeat.

More recently, these researchers followed up on their studies of relapse by observing people in a year-long behavioral weight-loss program and who were randomly assigned to either a low-calorie diet of 1,000 to 1,200 calories per day or a very low calorie diet of 400 to 500 calories per day.[29] Most people who put themselves on a moderate diet would eat more like the first group, so these dieters give us especially good information. In this research, the primary trigger for relapse differed between the two groups of dieters. Among the low-calorie dieters—people who ate similarly to those of us who go on moderate diets from time to time—emotions or moods were most often named as the primary triggers for their lapses: tension, anger, feelings of being down or rushed—notice the pattern of tense tiredness. But among the very restricted dieters, food and cravings were identified most often as the primary triggers. This result makes sense for people whose diets leave them well below their usual food intake. These people are starving.

I have argued that overeating occurs especially during periods of low energy and tension, and the relationship between diet relapses and extended low energy has been shown in research by David LaPorte at the University of Minnesota.[30] Studying obese women on very low calorie diets (420 calories per day) over ten weeks, he found that he could predict when diets would be broken by measures of anxiety taken once a week, but only during the second half of the study when a "fatiguing effect," as he called it, began to occur.[31] Similarly, weekly ratings of depression did not predict relapse until the last part of the study, but again, these women were more likely to eat when they were depressed once the fatiguing effect occurred. In other words, as the diet continued, physical resources declined and made it difficult for the dieters to withstand the hunger and bad moods.[32]

Depression

Depression is frequently identified as a cause of overeating. This makes sense because depression is characterized by low energy and increased tension, just the underlying pattern that motivates people to self-regulate with food. In several of the studies already described, feelings of depression were reported by dieters before they relapsed and as triggers for overeating. It is also true that serious depression often is associated with weight loss rather than gain, but weight loss is by no means the only outcome of serious depression as is evident by DSM-IV, the commonly used psychiatric classification system for Major Depressive Disorder.[33] There, a symptom of serious depression is *either* significant weight loss *or* weight gain and either a decrease or increase in appetite nearly every day. This tendency for either weight loss or weight gain is supported by empirical studies in which up to half of seriously depressed patients gained weight in the course of their condition.[34]

In any event there is little question that mood disorders are integrally related to eating problems. It is well known from a number of studies of so-called comorbidity, illnesses that exist together. And there is a close relationship between such eating disorders as anorexia and bulimia and mood disorders.[35] Other studies have shown correlations between binge eating and psychopathology, particularly depression,[36] and between depressive disorder and morbid obesity.[37] Still we may ask, just what is the relationship between depression and overeating? Does depression cause people to overeat or to eat less?

Several researchers believe that only some types of people gain weight when they are depressed, while others lose weight. Restrained eaters (dieters), obese individuals, and younger people are among those who have been identified as gaining weight when they are depressed.[38] I believe that another important reason for the differences is the degree of the depression.

Very depressed people may not even have the energy to eat. Less depressed people—those who experience feelings of depression from time to time—often use food as a self-regulator. It is quite possible that moderate depression stimulates overeating while serious depression can reduce eating. In the studies I described in which depression was distinguished as an eating trigger or as occurring before diet relapse, the depression identified was moderate in degree.

The last major trigger to overeating I will discuss is stress.

Stress

To understand the sometimes conflicting findings of researchers about the relationship between stress and overeating, we must consider different kinds of stress. One kind occurs when you have too much to do and too little time to do it. Perhaps you have ten urgent tasks but time to accomplish only five of them. With this scenario, you are constantly on the run. You don't think of anything other than the tasks and the hands of the clock. In this mode, food isn't a high priority; you just eat what you can. Junk food that is easily grabbed becomes a staple, and healthy diet is only a secondary consideration. When the pressures abate, and your energy is drained, food urges are common—usually for high-energy food.

Now think of a time that is less stressful, but one that still produces pressures and tense feelings. Maybe you have a demanding job. You don't have tight deadlines perhaps, but you are always busy and have many responsibilities. You might eat reasonably well; you are conscientious and try not to eat junk food. Nevertheless, you are frequently tempted to overeat by urges that dominate your consciousness, seemingly for no good reason. When these urges occur, all too often you succumb—usually when your resources are low—and the energy food you choose makes you consume more calories than you should.

With both kinds of stress you feel tension, a condition that motivates self-regulation. I have found in my studies that tension and stress are closely related, perhaps synonymous. One interesting point is that the same circumstances can be stressful at some times and not at others, and whether they are stressful depends on whether they cause tension. In other words, tension is a defining characteristic of a stress response. Why might the same circumstances be stressful sometimes and not others? It has to do with your energy level, with your physical resources. If you are very energetic, a demanding activity can be fun and stress free, but if you are tired the same activity can produce tension and stress.[39]

A third kind of stress is more extreme. Think of a middle-aged woman whom I will name Sara, who is experiencing a sudden and significant stressor because she just learned her husband is leaving her. She suspected a problem, but she didn't expect this, and she is devastated. Before hearing the bad news Sara had been reasonably well rested, she ate fairly well, and she was in good physical condition. Based on this healthy history, she did not deteriorate immediately when the stressful news came. With this kind of intense stress, however, certain predictable changes are likely to occur, some immediately and some over the course of a few days. It tends to cause a sharp increase in tension and an immediate draining of physical resources. In other words, it challenges what energy you normally have.

Over the next several days, Sara experienced insomnia as her physical resources declined and tension and fatigue (tense tiredness) began to dominate her mood. Stress of this kind will be most apparent at certain times of day, usually late afternoon and evening, times when daily energy cycles reach their natural low points for most people. Especially during these low-energy periods, but also at many different times of day, it was hard for Sara to concentrate on anything other than her unfortunate condition. Her work suffered. When she forgot her problems, the respite lasted only for a little while before distressing thoughts streamed back into her consciousness.

In the throes of this kind of stress, Sara tried to make herself feel better, but each time she tried to eat, she felt sick. With this high level of anxiety, some people turn to drugs or alcohol. Smokers may find themselves reaching for a cigarette more often than usual. Caffeine is another route, and the tension it can produce may make things even worse. Someone experiencing moderate stress might eat more, but Sara ate less and her weight continued to drop. At first she was pleased by her weight loss since she always had a problem with overweight, but soon it became apparent that it was making her unhealthy.

As you can see by considering these different kinds of stress, the problem of overeating is likely to be present with moderate stress, but intense stress can produce the opposite effect. This makes predicting how stress affects eating very difficult, and the scientific literature reflects this state of affairs. Then there is the problem of individual differences. Some of us react to stress by eating more and some don't.

There are quite a few published studies on stress-induced eating. It seems to me that one of the reasons scientists have focused so much on this relationship is a commonly held suspicion that when we go through prolonged periods of stress our personal habits lead us into unhealthy behavior. When we don't take care of ourselves well, we eat poorly. Sara wound up losing weight, but often stress results instead in weight gain. A recent study illustrates this pattern.

Stress and Food Choice

Andrew Steptoe and his associates in London studied sixty-nine male and female nurses and schoolteachers over an eight-week period.[40] These conscientious volunteers kept daily and weekly diaries in which they rated their degree of stress and mood as well as the hassles that affected them. From this it was possible to determine how much stress they were experiencing on a week-to-week basis. They also recorded their food and alcohol intake.

The findings give a good indication of how self-regulation occurs for a person under real-life stress. On stressful weeks, these people were significantly more tense, anxious, and depressed, and generally they rated their mood as more negative. In other words, the stress drove them to feel more tense and tired. During such weeks they ate significantly more fast food than during low-stress weeks.

Many stressful conditions make us tense and tired, and we naturally gravitate to foods that will replenish us and raise our energy. High-fat fast food accomplishes this, and is easy to get. A recent study at the University of Minnesota of the eating habits of over a thousand men and women showed that, among women, the frequency of eating fast-food meals was significantly correlated with energy intake and also with Body Mass Index.[41] In other words, those who ate more fast foods ate more energy-intensive food, and they weighed more. Looking at this correlation another way, you can predict how much people weigh by the amount of fast food they eat: more fast food, more weight.

In the English study, other self-regulatory behaviors were also in evidence. For example, alcohol consumption went up during high stress weeks, especially for those people who had indicated by questionnaire that they often drink to cope—an important individual difference. Another individual difference proved to be significant as well. Participants who had previously specified that food helps them to cope and cheers them up were significantly more likely to eat sweet food and also to eat cheese (a high-fat food) during the high-stress weeks. Finally men were likely to eat more red meat during high-stress weeks, while women were not.

What these nurses and teachers didn't do was exercise more during the high-stress weeks. This is perhaps understandable since exercise demands time, and stress often drains time. But, as we have seen, exercise is the single best way of coping with the tension and fatigue that inevitably result from stress.

Another study by Steptoe and his colleagues, indicated even more clearly how we eat to replenish our energy when we are under stress. In this research ninety retail sales workers were studied over a six-month period.[42] With this procedure the researchers were able to compare the weeks when the salespeople worked the most—more than forty hours a week—with weeks when they worked the least.

Again, it was found that these workers ate much more energy-intensive food—fat, sugars, and total carbohydrates— when they were under more stress. They were self-regulating their moods, seeking a way to increase their energy by using food. Other studies have duplicated these findings. We tend to compensate for our tension with high-calorie food.[43]

Who Eats More under Stress?

Individual differences have been the focus of research among psychologists for decades, and these kinds of studies have yielded valuable information about how some people are more likely than others to eat when they experience negative moods. What types of people are most vulnerable to overeating, how did they become more vulnerable, and what are the immediate circumstances that plunge them into overeating? These things obviously would be valuable to know, if for no other reason than that such individuals, once forewarned, could take special precautions. There is no unanimity among scientists about these differences, but I have some hypotheses that I will share with you.

Most studies have identified one type of person—the so-called restrained eater—as the most likely to overindulge when experiencing stress and negative moods. The profile of a restrained eater is a person who diets often and whose weight fluctuates frequently.[44] They are chronic dieters, and they have spawned a great deal of research.

One study illustrates this research nicely. Thomas Rutledge and Wolfgang Linden at the University of British Columbia in Canada recruited seventy-seven female undergraduate students and asked them to perform several stressful tasks during a twelve-minute period—mental arithmetic, a confusing perceptual task, and a word-scrambling function.[45] While filling out a questionnaire after completing these tasks, the subjects were told to help themselves to miniature chocolate chip cookies and snack crackers. The *real* behavior of interest was how much of these foods the women ate. Mood ratings also were made by the students, so the researchers could tell who was most affected by the stressful tasks. The restrained eaters who reported the most negative mood from the tasks were the most likely to eat the cookies and crackers. What this experiment appears to show is that dieters experiencing negative moods eat more.[46] More broadly and based on a number of other experiments, we can say that chronic dieters seem to act differently from others.[47]

I believe this is because of the heightened tension restrained eaters are under when they see attractive food—they must continuously be on guard against their urges to eat. When overeating has become a big enough problem to have led to chronic dieting, every possibility for overeating becomes a dangerous situation, which causes tension.[48]

With heightened tension, the process of self-regulation that drives many people to eat leaves these dieters especially vulnerable to overeating, the very temptation they are trying to avoid. Thus, any situation in which attractive food is salient—seeing television ads and supermarket displays, watching other people eating, and so on—is tension-inducing and becomes a stimulus for increased needs to self-regulate.

Although restrained eating is the most common individual difference that has been studied, a variety of other differences among types of people have been investigated through questionnaires.[49] Some vulnerable people apparently eat in response to external stimuli (such as attractive food) rather than internal cues such as hunger. Others experience a kind of disinhibition when they are under stress, taking drugs, or eating high-calorie foods, and subsequently they eat more. Then there are those who eat to counteract persistent and unusual hunger or who are attracted to particular foods. Also, some people appear to become depressed when they eat sugar, and this can set up a self-regulatory cycle of overeating. Finally, obese people are thought to be particularly vulnerable to overeating because of negative moods.

What these studies indicate is that people react differently to food, and some types of people in particular use it for more than just staving off hunger pangs. Because we are so different, I suggest that the best way to determine your own food habits and your reactions to food and stress is to keep a diary of when you are experiencing stress, tension and low energy. During these times, try to note what, how often, and how much you are eating. Only then will you understand why you overeat or why you can't stick with that diet.

Why Is Emotional Eating So Important?

All the hype and conflicting claims about overeating that bombard us daily in the popular media may confuse us and make it seem as though science provides no useful help with this universal problem. But that is not true. We may not as yet fully understand the genetics and the neurochemistry of overeating, but we do know that our moods often cause us to overeat—and moods can be managed. This fact offers real hope for those who struggle daily with problems of overeating.

It is clear that food is a comfort, something that makes us feel better. In times when we are feeling low or when we are stressed and frazzled, food can help. Why is this? Understanding the way drugs are sometimes used can aid in making sense of unhealthy food habits. Eating often is a kind of self-medication. And like other substances that can be used to self-regulate our moods, energy-intensive foods raise our spirits. They give us energy to deal with the tension we feel. Tense tiredness, the condition in which you feel both tension and fatigue, motivates us to eat, and sometimes to overeat. The evidence for this comes from a wide scientific literature on emotional eating. When properly understood you can see how our moods inexorably push us to become users, so to speak, but, in this case, users of the most universal drug of choice—food.

We have seen how urges to eat, the kind that break our well-planned diets, have apparent origins in tension and low energy. These feelings do not exist alone, of course. They are part of a larger complex of thoughts and habits, a complex that drives us first to think about a favorite food, often to obsess about it, and finally to eat too much of it. If the diet is broken, frequently there is a kind of snowballing effect that can push us into eating more than we need, and even into bingeing. Our moods are the key. When we eat, we feel better. Our tension is reduced and our energy is recharged, even if only in a subtle and temporary way.

This is how bad food habits form. The good feelings we experience after eating reinforce our behavior, and we want food when we experience even a small drop in energy or a little tension—whether or not we are hungry. And once we satisfy our feelings by eating, again we strengthen the learned behavior of overeating. Since much of the time we aren't even aware of how these bad habits work to guide our eating, we have little control over the pattern. We are bound to repeat the habits over and over again, no matter how much guilt we feel afterward.

One of the best ways of understanding overeating comes to us from studies of dieters who relapse, people who are committed to maintaining a certain diet but who succumb to inescapable temptations. And what are the conditions that led to their relapses? Once again, they are the moods that I have been talking about: tiredness, tension, depression, and feelings of being upset.

To escape the feelings, we try to self-regulate. We may use other words like "irritability," "weakness," or "constraint" to describe what happens just before the relapse, but they all describe this same state of tension and low energy. The pattern makes even more sense when we realize that relapses usually occur late in the day, in low arousal states, and when we are fatigued, hungry, and slightly tense.

Does Overweight Indicate Emotional Eating?

Negative moods exert powerful influences on our behavior, especially moods that are associated with tension and low energy. When our resources are depleted and our feelings of energy decline because of adverse life circumstances, we are often motivated to eat good tasting—energy-intensive—food as a way of feeling better. Eating can both raise our energy and reduce our tension. You can see this most clearly with the tense tiredness arising from stress or moderate depression and its influence on our desire for food, especially food that makes us feel better. Good-tasting food can give us resources for coping with negative moods, even if the resources are only temporary.

Our thoughts and behaviors are inexorably driven by eating habits when we are in the grip of these negative moods. These powerful influences may be stronger in some types of people than others, but for a large portion of the population negative moods cause overeating. Positive moods also can cause eating, of course, but in a different kind of way. In any event, our moods interact closely with our appetite and our tendency to eat.

To what degree is overweight specifically caused by our moods, as opposed to simple lifestyle habits of taking in more energy than is expended? Should the overweight person always look to emotional eating as a cause? As we gain unwanted weight or find it very difficult to take pounds off, should we blame our moods? And, if emotional eating is a cause of overweight, might we say that obese people commonly suffer from psychopathologies involving depression and anxiety?[50] The answers to these questions aren't certain, but the strength of the evidence about emotional eating together with the logic of the argument makes eating to regulate our moods one of the primary causes of overweight.

This is bound to be an unpopular idea because it appears to blame overweight people for their condition, implying that obesity is a kind of personal failing. It is much more popular nowadays to say that overweight is caused by uncontrollable factors such as heredity.[51] But the evidence for the influence of emotional eating is clear.

On the positive side, if overweight is caused by emotional eating, something can be done about it. Moods can be managed. This isn't as easy as taking some pills or eating more of a certain kind of food, but we know a great deal more about managing moods than we have ever known, so the battle against weight is winnable. Mainly, it takes understanding what is involved. This means understanding our moods.

We have seen how our moods and exercise are closely aligned and how our moods can drive us to overeating. We turn in the next chapter to the way obesity and simple overweight may be understood in relation to the balance between pleasure derived from food and pleasure from exercise. This is a basic biological equation for knowledge of how our bodies operate, and this knowledge can give us control over our weight—that elusive but reachable goal.

CHAPTER 5

Mood Pleasure

Food versus Exercise

WHEN YOU ARE LESS ACTIVE, you eat less, right? Actually, the answer is no; in many contexts the less active we are, the more we eat. This has a lot to do with why many of us are exercising less, eating more, and getting fatter and fatter.

Two classic studies on activity and food intake were conducted by Jean Mayer and his associates at the Harvard School of Public Health in the 1950s. The first, done with animals, showed that within a normal activity range, the more the animals were required to exercise on a treadmill, the more they ate.[1] This makes good biological sense, but over shorter periods of time, exercise did not increase appetite. And at the lowest activity levels, what the researchers called the sedentary range—the animals did not eat less, as might be expected. We can understand why animals would eat more as they become more active, but why would the least active animals eat more? It was an unexplained mystery.

Following up on the animal experiment, Mayer and his associates did a careful study of men working at a jute mill in India.[2] These workers lived away from home in the mill setting and had a very uniform diet, so it was possible to observe carefully how much they ate and to correlate that with their daily activity level. Once again, the workers with the most sedentary jobs—those whose jobs required them to sit at the shop all day or at their desks most of the time—ate more than many of the workers who were more physically active.

The question of why those who are least active would eat more remains unanswered. In modern-day society where many of us sit in front of computers all day, the answer would be especially relevant.

Pleasure from Food versus Pleasure from Activity

Some years ago my daughters and I spent a couple of days with some older relatives in Sweden, people in their seventies and eighties. They lived a sedentary life, without much physical activity. They treated us wonderfully and fed us the most sumptuous meals, and one of the things I noticed during that visit was that much of the conversation focused on the meals. Just after we finished one delicious meal and cleaned up the table, my relatives would begin to plan and talk about the next meal. In a certain respect these meals were the high points of their days, graciously offered to us. The pleasure they experienced each day seemed to be largely associated with food.

Since my daughters and I were used to much more physical activity than these relatives were, we would excuse ourselves between meals and go out to explore and hike in the countryside. Our high-energy times of the day were often spent hiking, although the meals, and especially the social interactions they provided, were most enjoyable. In other words, the pleasure we experienced each day extended beyond the meals to physical activity, as well as other things.

Since I try regularly to observe my own energy levels (an excellent index of all sorts of functions), I was struck by the fact that my daily high points—my most pleasurable times—often corresponded with my energy peaks, and as I observed my relatives, I became convinced that the same was true for them. The energy-generating meals of the day corresponded to their most pleasurable times. This no doubt came from the immediate energy they felt from the food as it was eaten, but certainly also from the preparation and planning, the general anticipation of the food. I believe that many people have similar reactions, and this is perfectly reasonable. After all, there is nothing wrong with having pleasure in your life, and there is nothing wrong with enjoying the pleasures of good food—so long as this enjoyment doesn't represent a disproportionate amount of the pleasure in your life or foster intense reactions.

Some time after the Sweden visit I discussed the matter in one of my classes, and afterward a young woman told me that she could understand perfectly how food could be the high point of my relatives' days. She was in her early twenties, and her weight didn't appear unusual. But the more we talked, the more clear it became that she had many "issues with food," as she called them. She probably had what would be described as an eating disorder, although it hadn't been diagnosed.

She said, for example, that she thought about food a lot. She told me how she could remember exactly what food she ate in restaurants during many past social interactions and, amazingly, what everyone else there ate as well. She realized that her attachments to food were a bit unusual and that they might not be good for her, but she had not made the connection between the pleasure experienced from food and the pleasure that might be experienced instead by physical activity. In my view, she had not focused sufficiently on how food is a disproportionate source of pleasure in her life, and on how the kind of pleasure she gets from food might be found instead in other activities.

Perhaps you can see how these ideas are related to mood from things I talked about in the last two chapters. In Chapter 3 I described the pleasure derived from exercise in relation to increased energy and decreased tension—mood elevation of a very basic sort. This mood reaction is an important part of the pleasure of movement. Physical activity, energy, and pleasure are integrally related, and this becomes especially apparent when you are deprived of activity. Anyone who has been temporarily incapacitated with an injury knows how excruciating the inactivity can be.

Forced inactivity is punishing, and this makes a great deal of sense within a biological perspective. From an evolutionary point of view, we know that our most important biological functions are highly rewarded, and they are maintained in many bodily systems so that they will endure.[3] Among the most vital biological functions is movement, because it enables us to transact our daily activities in relation to the subsistence of life. Thus, it makes sense that physical activity, energy, and pleasure are integrally related.

Feelings of pleasure from eating also are readily apparent, and these have a vital biological function as well. The pleasure from eating is especially present when you are hungry, but for many people this pleasure probably extends to all things associated with food. With hunger or appetite, however, these deficit states are associated with decreased energy and increased tension, the mood condition I call tense tiredness. So two vital biological functions, movement and eating, are both maintained to some extent by the pleasure that they produce. As we engage in these functions, the rewards that we experience ensure that the functions will continue. The pleasure is motivating. Of course, there are ways of feeling pleasure other than eating and physical activity, but these two are especially important for our topic because they relate to the basic equation of energy-in versus energy-out that maintains weight.

If eating is motivated in part by the pleasure that food produces, including increased energy and reduced tension, and if pleasure also comes from physical activity, again through increased energy and reduced tension, then to some degree one kind of pleasure can be substituted for the other. If the same basic mood states partially motivate you to eat and to exercise, then you should be able to self-regulate your moods with one or the other. And maybe exercising would produce fewer mood-driven food urges. It turns out that there is good scientific evidence showing exactly such a relationship. At least in the short term, exercise suppresses food urges, and this relationship offers potentially valuable tools for controlling appetite and maintaining weight.

Food, Pleasure, and Learning

How does the association between pleasure and the general constellation of food, food preparation, and food thoughts get formed? The answer to this question is necessary for understanding our basic orientation to food, as well as for understanding such things as overeating and overweight. To begin with, it is clear that the immediate effects of food often are feelings of pleasure. But what about energy feelings? These are probably influenced by increased blood sugar, as well as a host of other physiological activation changes that occur when we eat, although at present we don't know the exact physiological dynamics. Nonetheless, food is our main source of energy, and as such it can be expected to be closely tied to our most basic biological inclinations.

As we look carefully at how moods motivate us to eat, we can see not only that low energy is motivating but that when we are hungry, we are a bit tense as well. Food reduces our tension in a subtle way. The pleasure that food gives us is closely associated with increased energy and reduced tension, and, therefore, the way we self-regulate with food is motivated by avoiding the unpleasant feelings of tense-tiredness.

What about the larger constellation, including the preparation, anticipation, and thoughts about food? These things also can bring pleasure. They are, it seems to me, comparable to the salivation that Pavlov's dogs experienced in the famous laboratory studies of classical conditioning. His dogs learned an association between a sound and meat powder on the tongue, so eventually they salivated to the sound as well as to the meat. But they also salivated to the appearance of the handler, as well as other things associated with bringing the food. We have similarly learned to associate preparing, anticipating, and thinking about food with the pleasure of eating. We experience pleasure from these things because of conditioning, even when the food isn't present.

Learning affects our eating habits in many different ways. Take, for example, our attraction to good-tasting foods. It is as though our attention is drawn to them. Supermarket managers are well aware of how this works, and they stock all kinds of candy and sweets at the checkout line where we must wait to pay. If you doubt the Pavlovian conditioning effect, notice the next time you are looking at the candy that your mouth becomes moist, a kind of salivation. This is especially true if you are a little tired and tense. The pleasure you remember from eating candy in the past, including the mood effects that it produced, triggers all kinds of associations, and in this way you are motivated to eat, even when you don't need the food.

Compared to my Swedish relatives, my daughters and I had different learning histories and, consequently, different ways of self-regulating our moods. Our daily energy elevations —our daily pleasures—certainly came from the food we ate, as it did for everyone else, but the strong energy stimulus of physical activity was also important to us.

I suspect that some people have an intuitive understanding of these matters, even without knowing about the scientific principles involved. These are people for whom exercise and extended physical activity are an integral part of life. Much of the pleasure in their lives comes from physical activity rather than food. Moreover, I suspect they are people without significant food disorders.[4] These ideas about the balance of food and physical activity are not mysterious or difficult to grasp. But it is easy to lose sight of them.

Eating versus Physical Activity to Counteract Low Energy, Boredom, Anxiety, and Depression

Long-standing habits involving different kinds of balance between eating and physical activity tend to develop from many daily decisions. Consider, for example, sitting at home at night watching television, feeling increasingly tired (low energy), and seeking ways of staying awake before bedtime. Napping or sleeping might be the obvious remedy, but many people find that a nap in the evening leads only to disrupted sleep later. So you try other ways of remaining alert instead. Changing television programs to something more interesting, reading an exciting book, or doing some chores around the house are alternatives, of course. But for many people the choice is food. It gives you a certain amount of energy to stay awake.

Often the best alternative would be some light physical activity instead of food. As we saw in Chapter 3, getting up and moving around or taking a walk would counteract the tiredness immediately. Moreover, a short brisk walk leaves you more energized and more wakeful for some time, maybe an hour. More exercise later could do the trick again. But this requires effort, and your motivation to expend that effort is sapped by your tiredness. This kind of tiredness often comes from a lifestyle involving stress and lack of sleep.

Food, on the other hand, is a very easy way of counteracting the tiredness. And on top of that, it tastes good. You need only to walk a few steps to the cupboard or refrigerator and eat the good-tasting treat that will give you pleasure. Pose that against getting out of your chair and going for a brisk walk, and your tired thoughts about the two alternatives aren't even close: the cake wins, hands down! Many people make these kinds of decisions repeatedly, never realizing that they really have to do with managing energy. The decisions become habits, and the results are trim bodies or overweight ones.

We often forget that boredom is another stimulus to eating. Consider what boredom really is—a condition of tense tiredness, the state that I described as underlying negative moods. Notice the next time you are bored that you also feel slightly tense or jittery. You don't feel energized, except in a jittery kind of way. Scattered attention is a good indication of this. When you are tense you aren't good at focusing attention on mundane matters. Bored, you may surf through the TV channels looking for something that holds your attention, and often as not, you will be unable to find anything, since you are too tired and tense to remain attentive.

When boredom can't be reduced in other ways, food becomes the antidote for many people. It is the immediate cure for boredom. It raises your energy and dispels your tension—ever so subtly, but nonetheless reliably. Once again, physical activity is a wonderful alternative: it is an excellent tension reducer, and it gives you energy. Even a small amount of exercise can have a calming effect and, in turn, probably will reduce your boredom. But once again, eating often wins out; it is easier. For many people, long years of experience—a long learning history—assure that eating becomes the most attractive way of counteracting boredom.

Another example might be something troubling in your life that you can't stop thinking about. Each time you remember the problem you become slightly anxious, and, naturally, you seek to self-regulate in some way to eliminate that unpleasant feeling. Exercise, one of the best ways of reducing anxiety, is too often passed over for that immediate good-tasting treat. When you eat, your energy is increased and your tension reduced, and the unpleasant state of tense-tiredness is temporarily dispelled. Eating as a way of dealing with anxiety becomes habitual in the same way that the kind of eating caused by boredom becomes habitual. Through a simple learning process, you develop habits that gradually control you. The anxiety brings thoughts about good-tasting food and urges to eat something good. And it is a short step from thoughts and urges to eating the forbidden food. To control the habitual process, you must become aware of the way in which the mood-related eating is motivated.

Low-level depression is a well-known cause of overeating. And mild depression often goes unrecognized. The only signs may be tiredness, lack of energy, and no motivation to do necessary things. The energizing and tension-reducing effects of food are very attractive ways of self-regulating this condition. It is no wonder that overweight is so often the effect of mild depression. But exercise is also an obvious cure. It raises your energy and reduces your tension in a much more healthy way than unnecessary eating. Once again, when you are depressed there is a choice. Food is easy, but exercise is better.

These decisions to eat when you are tired, bored, anxious, or depressed may not be conscious. Usually you don't say to yourself, "I must stay awake, so I will eat something," or "I'm bored, and if I have that chocolate bar I won't be bored anymore." The feelings involved here are too subtle for people to be aware of them immediately, at least without some educated self-observation. Rather, eating when you feel that way is a habitual activity that has built up over many past experiences. Time and again in the past, you ate something and felt energized and less anxious. Then the same circumstances occurred anew, to be followed by further eating and further feelings of energy and calmness. This is the way habits develop. In a short time a pattern can be laid down in your brain that becomes automatic and that requires little or no conscious awareness. This lack of awareness makes it difficult to change. These conditioned reactions may seem like mysterious compulsions over which you have little control. But one of the things we have learned about habits is that, if you can become aware about how they operate, you can control them much more easily.

Understanding Weight Gain as Disproportionate Pleasure from Food

I hope it is apparent that the balance between energy-in and energy-out—which maintains our weight—has a very important basis in mood. If you self-regulate by seeking pleasure through food too much, there will be an imbalance and overweight will be the result. If you self-regulate by physical activity, healthy weight is more likely to occur. There may be variations on this theme that depend on differences in metabolism determined by our genes, natural set points, and so on, but the basic picture remains the same. And from this we can understand how people gradually gain weight.

A practical example occurred for me during a chance encounter at my university. Recently I spoke with a colleague who told me, "When I was twenty-five I weighed 160, and now that I am forty-three I weigh 190. I do pretty much the same things as I always did, but my weight keeps increasing." Does this sound familiar? It should because we tend to gain a pound or so each year as we get older.[5] When he said that he does pretty much the same things as he always did, I think that this is especially likely with regard to eating the same way, and the same amount. I suspect that he is not as physically active now as he was when he was twenty-five. Put this together with a natural slowing of his metabolism and you have a pre-scription for weight gain.

As I tactfully asked my colleague about his activity patterns, I learned that he used to enjoy pickup basketball games a couple of afternoons a week. Now he plays a slow game of golf, and only occasionally. I also reminded him that he used to park down the hill and walk to his office, but now he parks in a closer lot. "I know," he said defensively, "but I'm so busy I don't have time for the walk." As we further explored the matter of his decreasing activity, it became apparent that he isn't as active now as he was when he was younger in a variety of ways. Tiring of this conversation, he finally said, "Well, I am older now, so I don't have the energy I used to have." Exactly. He no longer has the energy reserves of his younger days, so he seeks energy in easy ways.

For my colleague, like most people as they get older, there is a gradu-ally shifting emphasis toward the pleasure and increased energy derived from food and away from the pleasure and energy of physical activity. To say this differently, the high points of his day are more likely to corre-spond to food as he gets older and less likely to correspond to physical activity. Overweight is the ultimate effect of this shift. This is a very likely explanation for why he weighs more now than he did nearly twenty years ago, and it is a good reason why most people gain weight as they get older.

What is the alternative? Increased physical activity. In fact, as you get older, as your metabolism slows and you process both food and physical activity less efficiently, you need *more* activity to maintain your weight, not less.

How Exercise Can Reduce the Urge to Snack

If one of the reasons we snack is for the pleasure it gives us in the form of increased energy and reduced tension, and if exercise also gives similar pleasure through its effect on our moods, then it ought to be possible to substitute exercise for snacking, at least in a limited sort of way. A few years ago, some of my students and I began to plan some experiments that would give us a better understanding of how this works. It seemed to us that we should be able to demonstrate that when the urge for a sugar snack hits, exercise could be used as a satisfying substitute. At the same time we could study the mood effects of eating and exercise to see whether they operate in the way I have suggested.

We designed a study to observe people who regularly eat candy, to learn whether their candy urge would be affected by exercise.[6] Eighteen male and female volunteers between eighteen and fifty-two years of age—all admitted sugar snackers—agreed to participate in this experiment, which lasted about three weeks.

On twelve different days, always at the same time and always after they had been sitting for at least forty minutes with no food or drink, they took out a candy bar and looked at it for a few seconds to stimulate their urge. Then they rated the strength of that urge on a seven-point scale. They also rated their energy and tension using a mood checklist that I developed some years ago.[7] Following the ratings, they either took a brisk five-minute walk or they remained seated and continued doing what they had been doing for five more minutes.[8] Then they rated their appetite and mood a second time. With this procedure we were able to compare their urge to eat the candy after walking with the urge after sitting.

The striking results confirmed our hypotheses. After walking briskly for five minutes, their urge for the candy decreased, but after sitting their urge actually increased. Apparently, viewing the candy bar had done its trick, and after sitting for five minutes our subjects wanted the candy even more. At the end of five minutes of walking, however, they wanted the candy less than they had just five minutes earlier. These differences were statistically significant.

There was another interesting result of this experiment that was quite telling. After our subjects had done the second ratings, they were free to eat the candy whenever they wished. But they were required to make note of how many minutes elapsed before they ate it. It turned out that those who had walked waited almost twice as long to eat the candy bar than those remaining seated—nearly twenty minutes compared to almost ten minutes—and sometimes they didn't even eat the candy after walking. The urge to eat the candy was decreased by the exercise.

The mood ratings revealed other things as well. Energy feelings were increased significantly, and feelings of tension were decreased significantly, by the walking compared to sitting. This small amount of exercise shifted the participants' mood toward what I call calm energy. In this mood state food urges are not nearly as common. Compare this to the unpleasant tense tiredness that motivates people to self-regulate, often with food.

Think about this experiment the next time you are sitting around feeling the urge for something sweet to eat. These urges come and go, and if you can withstand them for a little while, that's often all you need to avoid them.

If you are skeptical, try the experiment yourself. The next time that you have an urge to eat, but it isn't because you haven't eaten for a while and need food, rate your urge, take a short brisk walk, and then notice whether you have the same urge. If you find that your urge diminishes right after the walk, this will be extremely valuable information for you. I'm not suggesting that you can do away with all unwanted food urges in this way because the mood effect tends to be temporary, but this knowledge may help you understand why you have these urges and potentially how you might begin to deal with them.

Other research has also shown that exercise temporarily suppresses appetite, although in those experiments scientists did not study the underlying moods the way we did, and they concentrated on standard meals rather than sugary snacks. For example, in two studies at the Human Appetite Research Unit at the University of Leeds in England, subjects came to the laboratory in the morning, ate breakfast, and then stayed there until mid-afternoon.[9] After breakfast the participants either pedaled an exercise bike or sat and read. The researchers were interested in how much energy was expended during twenty-seven minutes of fairly intense exercise (70 percent VO_2 max) or sixty minutes of light exercise (30 percent VO_2 max), and they periodically collected expired air to test it. While the experimental participants were at the research unit, they rated their hunger and their desire to eat several times, and for lunch they were allowed to help themselves to sandwiches, fruit cocktail, strawberry yogurt, and biscuits. They ate lunch about noon but they could eat earlier if they wanted to, and the time they chose to eat was recorded. For the rest of the day and the next morning, the participants kept food diaries so researchers could determine whether the exercise had increased their food intake.

The findings were very much the same as in our research. Both hunger and desire to eat were decreased by the exercise, particularly the more intense exercise. The suppression of hunger lasted for over an hour, but its greatest effect was fifteen minutes following the exercise. Moreover, following the exercise the participants delayed eating compared to the control condition, when they read. In another technical analysis of the energy that was expended by the exercise and the amount that was eaten, the researchers were able to demonstrate further appetite suppression for the rest of the day by showing that there was a negative energy balance because of the exercise, but the participants did not eat more.

The research I described and other somewhat similar experiments[10] clearly suggest that exercise can suppress appetite, and this information is extremely valuable for practical use. You can use exercise as one tool for appetite suppression, especially during those periods of low mood that occur periodically each day. These studies provide clear support for the observation that food and exercise balance each other and that one underlying reason has to do with the way mood influences the two.

Appetite, Hunger, and Their Cause in Physiology and Mood

Are there explanations other than mood for the way exercise suppresses appetite? We know that hunger probably has a complex physiological basis, and although scientists are not certain how hunger arises, the origins of hunger sensations are likely to be found in the brain, gut, liver, adipose tissue, and endocrine hormones.[11] Careful experiments show that changes in one or more of these systems influence eating. I believe, however, that moods are like signal systems of these underlying processes. They tell us about basic physiological conditions that are occurring, and they motivate us to take action. In the case of hunger, the feelings of low energy and tension arise from these physiological deficits, and they motivate us to eat.

So, do our moods cause us to eat? Cause and effect is a complicated relationship to prove in this case. For the first causes, of course, basic physiological processes are at work. But our moods represent conscious information about these physical processes. As conditions of hunger arise from physiological deficits, we experience negative feelings that we interpret as low energy and tension. When we feel this way we are often motivated to eat as a way of changing these negative feelings—negative feelings are strong motivators. The mood that occurs from exercise involves similar systems, but in a positive way. Exercise affects the body in a wide variety of complex patterns, including a kind of general arousal that parallels the arousal that occurs from food ingestion. The elevated moods that we experience from exercise are inconsistent with the negative moods that motivate us to eat and, with this, appetite is suppressed through moderate exercise.

The strong influence of moods is evident in a distinction that scientists make between hunger and appetite. *Hunger* sometimes is used to refer to the more basic biological state that is driven by nutritional deficits, in distinction to *appetite*, which includes all kinds of psychological associations. Such influences as food choices, conditioned reactions, and preferences for specific tastes and nutrients all contribute to appetite. Here mood is likely to be particularly influential.

Appetite Suppression and Mood: The Wider Circle of Evidence

A variety of substances can suppress appetite. Generally these arouse or activate us. For example, it is well known that cocaine and amphetamine can temporarily suppress appetite, and sometimes this is the motivation for their use.[12] A good example of this is Camryn Manheim, the popular Emmy-winning star of the television program *The Practice*. She has recently become a worthy spokesperson for overweight women, and in an interview for *Parade* magazine admitted taking crystal methedrine to lose weight.[13] This amphetamine-like substance, sometimes known as "speed," produces mood changes comparable to those of various kinds of diet pills, although often much stronger. The drug helped her drop 80 pounds, but the health effects of losing weight this way are dangerous.

Cocaine and amphetamine aren't the only activating substances that suppress appetite. Other, more widely used drugs such as nicotine and caffeine appear to suppress appetite temporarily as well. Nicotine has the paradoxical effect of both activating and relaxing the smoker. This doesn't make sense unless we understand that nicotine activates by raising energy and relaxes by reducing tension—two central mood effects.[14] One interesting thing about this mood change is the effect it has on appetite. It is a well-known phenomenon that many people who stop smoking subsequently gain weight. It now seems clear how this could happen. In one study, Sharon Hall and her associates at the University of California, San Francisco, put people on a program in which they stopped smoking at different times. Whenever they ended their cigarette use, their ingestion of sucrose and fats increased proportionately.[15] Without the lift and relaxation that the cigarettes provided, the smoking abstainers apparently turned to an alternate mood regulator—food.

Recall the way exercise elevates mood and also suppresses appetite. With nicotine we have a similar appetite suppression, and even though some different systems of the body are involved, the mood effects appear to be the same. Both exercise and nicotine raise energy and reduce tension. Once again, you can self-regulate by food, smoking, or exercising. In all these cases mood is what is being self-regulated.

The appetite-suppressing effects of diet pills usually are explained in terms of how they influence the brain through the biochemistry of catecholamines (for example, norepinephrine) or through serotonin, although there is no certainty about exactly how this works to reduce appetite.[16] But various types of diet pills have common mood effects, and these may be an important reason why they suppress appetite. Take, for example, the well-known appetite-suppressing drug combination known as fen-phen. This drug worked well in helping people to lose weight until it was taken off the market because it could potentially cause heart damage. In one study of fen-phen that Lisa Brauer and her associates at the University of Chicago conducted, they found that one of the constituents, phentermine, energized people in a similar way to amphetamine.[17] The other constituent, fenfluramine, activated people by increasing their tension. This would not normally be seen as a mood elevator, but as we shall learn in the next chapters, when tension is paired with increased energy the overall mood effect can feel good. In any event, taken as a combination, the ingredients in fen-phen suppressed appetite.

If both appetite suppression and mood elevation occur from exercise, nicotine, amphetamines, and fen-phen, could mood be the reason that they all reduce eating? Do people eat less because they do not need to self-regulate with food when their mood is elevated in any of these ways? I think that they do.

Adjusting the Balance Between Food and Physical Activity

Have you ever been dismayed when you caught an unexpected view of yourself in the mirror, or become distressed when you noticed that your clothes were too tight, or you were just reminded that your weight is increasing when you stepped on a scale? For a great number of us, this is a very unpleasant reality. The more than $30 billion a year that Americans spend on controlling their weight is a testament to our motivation to do something, sometimes desperately, about this state of affairs.[18] The lucky few can eat whatever they want with no effect, and often creeping weight gain isn't true for the young, with their well-functioning metabolisms. Women are more likely to be troubled about high weight than men, but in today's shape-conscious society it is a problem for the vast majority. When there is a change in weight, it means that the balance between food and physical activity is shifting. Let's think about how this works.

Earlier I mentioned a colleague who used to weigh 160, but nearly twenty years later, weighs 190. He probably eats the same, but as he's aged, his activity level has decreased. The decline in physical activity as people grow older is well documented.[19] And a recent U.S. Surgeon General's report makes this perfectly clear when it shows, from several large studies, that leisure-time physical activity declines with age.[20] One well-known study seemed to counter this pattern when it showed a shift toward greater activity in men after age sixty-five (probably as retirement allowed them to be more active),[21] but for the most part, gradually lessening physical activity is true for most people as they grow older.

Although physical activity patterns decline with age, we tend to develop habits for how many meals and how much food per meal we eat, and these remain the same even though we need less food energy with declining physical activity. An interesting point here is that such a disparity can occur only with relative affluence. In primitive societies where resources are scarce, the old eat less even as they produce less. If we look at our own society, a moment's consideration about how this shifting balance might be corrected leaves us two choices: more activity or less food.

While age is a common general explanation for the gradually shifting balance between food and physical activity, declining mood is another important and related reason. Mood shifts can occur because of changes in life circumstances that lead to increased stress, low-level depression, compromised health that reduces physical activity, or, in general, any change that reduces energy and increases tension over time. If you notice that your weight is gradually creeping up, pay attention to important things that commonly put you in a bad mood—lack of sleep, chronic personal problems, health problems and muscle aches that restrict activity, pessimism about your future, and a host of other reasons for declining energy and increasing tension.

Not only do these slowly changing life circumstances shift the balance between exercise and food, but as we gain weight our energy is depleted. Twenty-five extra pounds is like carrying around a grocery bag of canned goods all the time—not to mention declining self-esteem about being unable to master the weight problem. As Oprah Winfrey once said when she had lost a great deal of weight, "Losing weight was the single greatest achievement in my life."[22] Inability to control one's weight can be a severe threat to self-esteem and can result in giving up and choosing the easiest route to energy—food.

Up until now I have spoken in a general way about moods and about underlying differences in energy and tension as the bases of our moods. Now it is time to examine these elusive states more carefully. There are thousands of scientific studies that allow us to understand the origins as well as the management of everyday moods, and we turn to these topics next. Our moods are so basic to our lives that they influence, at least in some way, almost all aspects of our daily behavior. In the preceding pages I have argued that controlling overeating starts with understanding and then managing your moods, but, as we shall see, the influence of moods is much wider than that. In the next chapters we will begin to examine how.

CHAPTER 6

Why Do We Have Moods?

HI, JANET. HOW ARE YOU?" I said as we waited for our sandwiches
at a food counter at my university. "I'm in a bad mood," she told
me with a tight voice. She talked quietly so that others wouldn't
hear.

"Why?" I said.

"Well, you're the expert, so you tell me," she said with a forced grin.

Janet, an excellent and very conscientious administrator, is in her early
forties. She was aware of my books on mood; in fact, she told me that she
had purchased one of them, but hadn't read it yet. I asked her what had
been happening in her life lately. I could see the tension in her face, and I
realized that her voice sounded more pinched than usual.

"Oh, we're preparing a budget and we have a new system with complicated software that doesn't seem to work right," she said. "And, of
course, the budget has to be ready yesterday." She then told me that she
had been working from early morning to late at night, getting too little
sleep, and eating sandwiches or other fast foods when she had time to
grab something.

I said, "Well, you know, too little sleep is a very important reason for
being in a bad mood because our moods are linked to energy and tiredness, and lack of sleep is one of the most degrading influences on energy."
Seeing that she wanted to hear more, I mentioned that the present time of
day—it was three o'clock—could be another important reason for the
bad mood. When we are under stress, I said, we get more tense as energy
sinks in its natural daily cycle, and mid- to late afternoon is a low energy

point for many people. I also referred to the way that *not* eating is important to our moods. (It was a late lunch for both of us.) With that, she shook her head vigorously as though she felt vaguely guilty about her current diet. (I noticed that she had a big bag of chips and a large cup of coffee along with her sandwich.) Finally, I gave her some reassuring words by saying that an informal survey about mood I took in a couple of senior-level psychology classes showed that bad moods last only about half a day on the average.[1] (Good moods last longer.)

The Measurement of Mood

Mood is a hot topic in current scientific research. Thousands of articles and books have been published about mood in the past ten years. The reason that moods are included in the category of emotional states is that moods are like emotions, although longer in duration and usually less intense.[2] Lesser intensity isn't always the case, however, as anyone in the grip of an intense depression is well aware. Also, unlike emotions, moods somehow tend to be more mysterious in the sense that they seem to come and go for unexplained reasons, whereas emotions often have causes that we understand.

If a vicious dog lunges at you, fear will be the emotional effect of this cause, but your feelings probably will dissipate after a short while. On the other hand, if you are feeling tense and fearful the next day, but you have forgotten the dog, we would call this a negative mood. Even if the dog were the initial cause of your feelings, chances are that if those feelings lasted into the next day they have been influenced by something other than the dog. The causes of our moods are not nearly so mysterious as many people think once some basic principles are understood, and I will review many of those principles here.

A couple of comments about terminology and measurement are in order before we begin. The term *affect* is employed sometimes in medical and scientific language, and often it is used in a roughly synonymous way with *mood*.[3] Affect is often a surface feeling, though, while mood is a longer-lasting state. Reflecting the transitory nature of affect as the term is used in psychiatric circles, clinical psychologists or psychiatrists may speak of a patient's affect in relation to crying, laughing, or ways of talking, and you can hear such terms as "labile affect" for rapidly changing emotional reactions that are symptoms of some psychiatric conditions.

We often find *affect* and *mood* used interchangeably in scientific research, and here almost always there is some description by the person of how he or she feels, usually with reference to a mood checklist. An absence of this vital knowledge concerning how the individual feels, by the way, is one of the major weaknesses in research with animals, and animal research is used almost exclusively by many scientists to try to understand the biochemistry of moods. Thus, rats are used in most research when scientists are trying to assess biochemical changes in the brain, but these animals obviously can't tell us what mood they are in—if, indeed, they even do have moods.

Research on humans usually records the immediate feelings as the subject rates them, or the person is asked how he or she felt in the past hour, day, or week. Self-rated moods often are correlated with other variables—for example, moods just before there is an urge to eat junk food. Incidentally, people without significant psychological problems are fairly good at describing their current moods, but descriptions of how they felt earlier in the day or on previous days have less accuracy.[4]

The most common way of measuring mood in scientific research on humans is to ask the experimental subject to read a list of mood-descriptive adjectives and to rate his or her current feelings on each adjective. So, for example, we might ask, "At this moment how *depressed/happy/energetic/tense* do you feel?" The most commonly used measure of normal moods is an adjective checklist called the *Profile of Mood States* or *POMS*.[5] Another common mood measure is one I developed some years ago that is especially used by scientists when biological or physiological correlates of moods are of interest. This is called the *Activation-Deactivation Adjective Check List (AD ACL)*.[6]

How Many Moods Do We Have?

Counting and classifying are the primary activities in developing the science on a particular subject. For example, biologists made great advances in understanding plants and animals with the development of the phylogenetic scale. With this classification system, they are able to see similarities and common ancestries of various species, for example. In a somewhat similar way, in studying moods there has been a great deal of research to develop a classification system to try to learn the answers to such questions as how different moods are related to one another, whether there are common causes of different groupings of moods, and even how many moods there are. This research usually starts with adjective checklists.

The foremost pioneer in this area was Vincent Nowlis, a now-retired professor at the University of Rochester (and my doctoral dissertation professor.)[7] Nowlis set out to measure many different kinds of moods by constructing complex adjective checklists that contained all the different moods that could be identified. Large numbers of people then rated their current moods with these checklists, and with these self-ratings he used a mathematical-statistical procedure called *factor analysis* to determine whether a small number of factors or dimensions accounted for all the moods that the adjectives represent. In this way he sought to learn how many moods there are and how the different moods or feelings that we have are related. One conclusion he reached was that there are twelve separate dimensions of mood—in other words, twelve basic ways that people experience moods: aggression, anxiety, surgency, elation, concentration, fatigue, social affection, sadness, skepticism, egotism, vigor, and nonchalance. The *POMS,* developed in large part from Nowlis's research, includes the dimensions of tension-anxiety, vigor, fatigue, and confusion-bewilderment.

Speaking of the last dimension in the *POMS,* you may be confused and bewildered at the many different moods that scientists have discovered. You may say, "All I know is that I'm either in a good mood or a bad mood," or that sometimes you are depressed or happy or you just feel pleasure, and that's the way you think about moods. Scientists working in this area have tried to understand these basic kinds of feelings.

My own research on moods took Nowlis's work into account, but I was especially interested in the biological bases of moods. It seemed to me that there were a smaller number of more basic biopsychological dimensions of moods than the twelve that Nowlis identified. I used similar mathematical procedures, such as factor analysis, but I also paid attention to more general biological variables like daily biological rhythms related to alertness and tiredness and the effects of such things as exercise, food, and stress.

Over many years my research kept showing that most of the different kinds of moods we experience, day in and day out, have in common two basic biopsychological dimensions. One of these I named *Energetic Arousal,* or Energy for short, and the second I named *Tense Arousal,* or just Tension. You can see from Figure 6.1 how these two dimensions are related and you can see some other terms that I coined to talk about variations of the two. The common moods that most people think about are related to energy and tension. Really good moods have high energy and low tension (calm energy), and bad moods such as depression tend to have low energy and high tension (tense tiredness). Pleasure and happiness tend to be associated with calm energy, while despair is associated with tense tiredness. Incidentally, strong urges to eat when we don't really need the food are related to tense tiredness as well.

During the last twenty years or so a great deal of other research has been done, and other classification systems have been proposed. Research on moods has been less weighty and not as well publicized as some well-known systems in biology, but in many ways seeking the basic dimensions of mood has been like the search for the structure of DNA that resulted in discovery of the double helix.

As an example of some of the other systems proposed to understand mood, James Russell and his students and colleagues at the University of

FIGURE 6.1

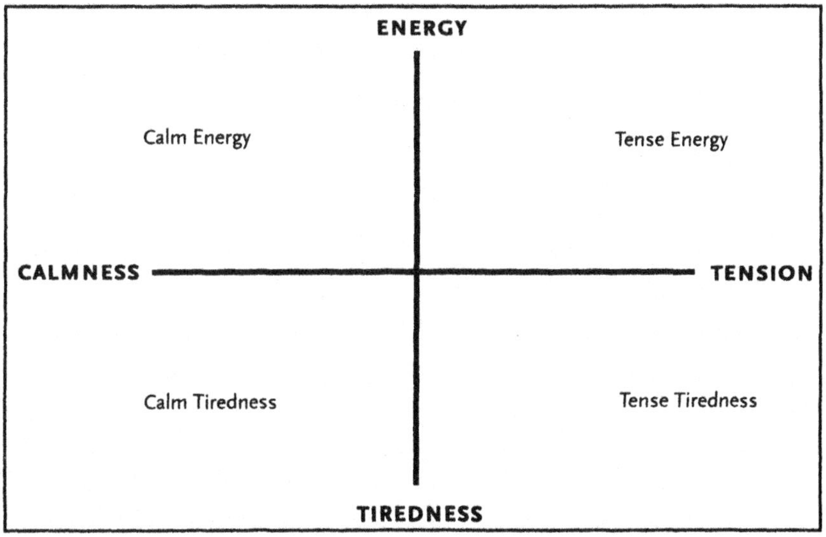

Source: Robert E. Thayer, *The Origin of Everyday Moods* (New York: Oxford University Press, 1996)

British Columbia argue that the basic dimensions of moods are two that he calls *Pleasure* and *Arousal* (later known as *Activation*).[8] The moods represented by Russell's dimensions are roughly the same as the mixtures of moods that range from calm energy to tense tiredness and from tense energy to calm tiredness. In other words, we agree about the dimensions, but we call them different names and we differ slightly over what feelings are included in the dimensions. Most important, we differ in what dimensions are most basic: energy and tension or pleasure and activation.

Another classification system is one developed by James Watson and Auke Tellegen at the University of Minnesota, in which the basic dimensions are called *Positive Affect* and *Negative Affect*,[9] later renamed *Positive Activation* and *Negative Activation*.[10] A great deal of research has been done on correlates of these two dimensions, and they are quite well known. These two dimensions are almost identical to what I call Energetic and Tense Arousal, respectively, and this may be one of the reasons that they recently renamed their dimensions. This similarity is not surprising since Watson and Tellegen developed their dimensions by combining and re-analyzing my research results as well as the results of others. Positive and Negative Affect differ from mine primarily by how they relate to each other, a point I will go into in more detail in the next chapter. Variations of these mood dimensions have been put forward by other researchers as well.[11]

What Underlies Good and Bad Moods?

Calm Energy

In your best moods you feel energetic, and at the same time, there is an absence of tension: calm energy. The highly conditioned athlete who is brimming with energy, but calm at the same time, often experiences this mood. Incidentally, in studying world-class athletes, exercise scientists have coined the term "iceberg profile" to refer to a state of high vigor and low negative moods—a kind of calm energy.[12] Other states that probably are underlaid by calm energy include what some people call *Flow* and the *Zone,* although to my knowledge specific mood research indicating calm energy has not been done on these states. In Eastern culture, the Zen master presumably experiences calm energy in much of life. This individual engages in normal daily activity, but with perfect calmness.[13]

But what is the experience of energy without tension really like? Think about being both energetic and calm at the same time. It's a very special state. With this mood, nothing bothers you greatly and you aren't hurried; yet you are ready to do things: to work, to play, to run errands, to sit and talk to someone with undivided interest and enthusiasm. Not being tired, you aren't yawning and wishing you could sleep. With calmness, you avoid wondering what time it is and how long this is going to take you. You aren't nervous in any way, and there is an absence of the muscle tension in your body and face that would arise with stress, fear, or anxiety. Energy without tension weds us completely to the situation at hand. Our attention is completely focused. If a number of things have to be done, we do each in its turn without continually thinking about what's next. We have the ability to choose our activities in an unhurried fashion. Given the option, we want calm energy and seek it, and this is the reason we self-regulate to be in this state. Calm energy is patient and attentive, productive, and pleasant. In our research we find that people rate this state as the most pleasant of the mood combinations. I think of it as underlying our most optimal moods.

When I speak to groups about calm energy, I often get a response from individuals who don't quite understand energy without tension. They say something like, "When I feel energetic I always feel a little wired or tense at the same time. Isn't that the way it is for everyone?" Today, with stress on the rise, most people are a little tense much of the time, and for them calm energy may be so unfamiliar as to seem nonexistent. Some are very familiar with calm energy, however. People who have meditated a lot, or practiced yoga, or those who regularly use other stress-management techniques know immediately what I mean. Even deep prayer as a kind of meditation practice often leads to calm energy. Athletes are familiar with this state, probably because the vigorous exercise they undergo produces relaxation and calmness mixed with increased energy.

Calm energy relates in predictable ways to seeking physical activity and following sensible eating practices. Since exercise feels good, when we have energy we seek it out. We may look forward to a good workout, or just a leisurely walk, and stress is no problem when we feel calm, so time is not a limitation on our activity. Moving about, walking, or exercising our muscles brings pleasure; therefore, with calm energy physical activity is not avoided. Calm energy also gives us a more intelligent feeling about what food we need. As our energy gradually declines and food is necessary for replenishment, for example, we eat what we need and no more. Our food choices tend to be best for optimal physical replenishment, and not based on tension-driven urges and appetites. We want what is necessary for the immediate needs of our body, but when our resources are replenished we stop eating. With calm energy, overeating is not a problem.

Nick, the owner of popular deli in Seal Beach where I live, is a man I associate with an active kind of calm energy. Everyone likes Nick, partly because of his infectious energy, a kind of up-beat active state of mind. Although he is usually quite busy, his mood is without any obvious nervousness or tension. He does each task completely as it is required, but even with his thriving business you always have the sense that he is completely attentive to the task at hand, completely involved in your interaction with him while it is occurring. In other words, he doesn't seem distracted.

Most would think of Nick as happy, and he makes others who deal with him a little happy as well. Nick is forty-eight, five foot nine, and 173 pounds. He is not a bit overweight, and, except for his mood, this might be surprising because he loves food and he knows all about it. He plays racquetball regularly and, while he enjoys food greatly, he does not overeat. He probably is a man blessed with good genes, but I am convinced that his demeanor of calm energy is an important reason for his healthy associations with food and exercise.

Tense Energy

While calm energy may underlie the best moods, good moods also may involve some tension as well as energy. I call the mood in which the two are combined tense energy. This often is your mood when you are extremely busy, but at the same time very productive. Tense energy regularly occurs at late morning, for example, when you have lots of work that must be done in a short period of time, but you are healthy, you had a good night's sleep, and you ate a nutritious breakfast. You might think of this state as revved up and clicking on all cylinders. In our research we find that people often rate tense energy as a positive feeling. You can accomplish lots of work in this state (although, as we will see later, your highest-quality work probably comes with calm energy).

Tense energy is sometimes used for motivation. I occasionally joke about some of my procrastinating students who wait until the last minute to study for an exam, or begin to write a paper the night before it is due. The tension that they feel in the last minute is born of fear of failure, and if that tension isn't too great, it energizes them. It gets them going, and it motivates them. Tense energy probably is the predominant state of Type A personalities, and so-called Type T personalities, or thrill seekers. These people appear to enjoy being on the edge.[14]

Tense Tiredness

The worst moods are underlaid by tense tiredness. This is the state that occurs when your resources are depleted and at the same time you feel tense, anxious, or nervous. Depression, for example, involves low energy and either moderate or high levels of tension.[15] The previously described state of tense energy may be a pleasant one in which you get a lot done, but it depends on at least a moderate amount of energy, and energy dissipates as your resources decline. If you are under stress, and tension remains high, the decline in energy that inevitably occurs leads to the unpleasant state of tense tiredness and to all sorts of moods that we describe as bad or negative.

If you ever have experienced chronic tension—and, in this day and age, most of us have—you may have realized that at the same time you were tense, your resources still varied up and down with different amounts of sleep, food, and exercise. In other words, your energy was sometimes high and sometimes low while you felt tense. From this, you can get a basic understanding of when bad moods occur: they are times when you feel tense and simultaneously low in energy. For example, if you are predisposed to feelings of depression, it is easy to see when these feelings will appear. Similarly, people tend to have food urges and they may overeat when they feel tense and tired. Again, you can predict those times just by recognizing your tension and your changing levels of energy. Tense tiredness often leads to overeating.

A woman called into a radio program on moods where I appeared as a guest expert and gave a typical scenario in her description of a hectic day at work.[16] She indicated that she puts out a magazine and in the first two weeks of the month has to work as efficiently as possible and to maintain a very high level of energy. During those two weeks, she said, she works until she gets tired, then she sleeps until she wakes up, and then she works again until she gets tired (about three or four hours of sleep at night and some sleep in the daytime). She went on to describe a problem she has with food. Giving up cigarettes was not difficult for her, she said, but food was another matter. She suggested that poor eating habits were like an unbreakable addiction in her life.

This woman undoubtedly experiences tense energy alternating with tense tiredness and exhaustion much of the time when she is working on a hectic schedule. During the high energy times, I suspect that she would describe her moods as reasonably pleasant and with no particular problems. But a natural tendency to self-medicate—to reduce the bad mood—coupled with unhealthy food choices when feeling tense energy probably leads to overweight. The stress of constant work, little sleep, and the demand for high energy drives her to seek energy through food. It's highly likely that her time demands leave her feeling that she cannot stop work to benefit from the natural antidote to stress: exercise.

Calm Tiredness

Calm tiredness, another way that energy and tension are experienced in our bodies, often occurs late in the day and especially when there is not much stress. For example, if you are on a vacation, or maybe a relaxing weekend, as your energy declines toward evening, you can fully experience this state of calm tiredness. Like calm energy, this also can be a pleasant state—in other words, a good mood. In our research we find that people rate calm tiredness as positive, but not as positive as calm energy. As your energy declines in its natural cycle toward nighttime, the absence of tension can lead to a very pleasant and deep sleep. But if tension remains even moderately high, you can expect insomnia. Or when you do go to sleep, you can expect fitful and unsatisfying sleep. Calm tiredness, on the other hand, produces, as we say, the deep sleep of the gods.

Happiness

Happiness is the topic of a good deal of psychological research and receives a lot of media attention.[17] The immediate feeling of happiness is most closely associated with calm energy. In fact, in careful psychometric research we find that when people rate themselves as happy at the moment, they also rate themselves as more energetic and less tense.[18] We all feel happy and sad from time to time, but scientists also find that happiness is associated with longer-lasting personality *traits*. For example, people who describe themselves as commonly happy tend to be high on the trait of extraversion and low on the trait of neuroticism.[19] On this more general level, happiness—or subjective well-being, as it is sometimes called—is predicted by personality as well as by good health and higher socioeconomic levels.[20] But whatever the more enduring influences on a happy life may be, the immediate experiences of happiness usually occur during states of calm energy.[21]

Anger

Basic emotions such as anger and sexual arousal are also associated with the biopsychological mood dimensions I have described. Both anger and sexual arousal involve heightened energy and varying degrees of tension, either tense energy or calm energy. But researchers differ in their viewpoint on these matters. One of the things that indicates to me the importance of energy in anger is that you are less likely to be angry when you are very fatigued, although you may experience short bursts of anger. You may have noticed as well that if there is a cause for anger, your feelings are stronger when you are energized. If you are angry and you begin to exercise—a common way of increasing energy—you will become more angry, at least until the exercise tires you out. If you are angry but you are holding your anger back, tension definitely is present, as well as energy. On the other hand, unrestrained anger may involve little tension.

Although anger appears to be related to energy on a momentary level, when anger is judged over time—for example, the angry personality—it is related to other negative emotions of fear, sadness, and shame.[22] Thus people who are angry much of the time also tend to be fearful and sad during extended periods. Although the exact relationship between anger and mood is not agreed upon by all researchers, I believe that on a momentary level it is most closely related to energetic arousal, but depending on circumstances, tense arousal also may play a part. This conclusion makes the most sense from a biological perspective, since anger facilitates striking out or aggressing, and, unlike fear, this "action tendency" is most facilitated by energy.

The old psychoanalytic theory of catharsis is an interesting case in relation to anger and energy. Researchers have found that catharsis doesn't seem to work much of the time.[23] Expressing anger often leads to more anger, not less. The expression of anger energizes you, and that in turn leaves you ready for a bigger fight. But I believe that in one respect the principle of catharsis probably does hold, and that is when your angry outburst is sufficiently taxing that it finally exhausts you. In any event, if the cause of your anger hasn't been resolved, chances are that the next time the same cause is present you may become angry again, and therefore catharsis hasn't really been effective.

As you may recall from Chapter 4, anger is one of the emotions that often is described as occurring before overeating. This is an interesting point because, unlike the usual states that lead to overeating—such as depression—anger appears to involve high energy. Why would we seek food, an energy elevator, when we are already in a state of high energy? The answer isn't clear, but I believe that we don't eat at the height of our anger, but rather just after the peak, when some fatigue sets in. Another possibility is that the energy of anger overcomes any inhibitions we may have, including dietary inhibitions. Then, of course, there is the Freudian possibility that by eating we can punish those who disapprove of our weight. More research is necessary before answers to these motivational questions are known.

Sexual Arousal

In a similar way to anger, sexual arousal is reduced by tiredness and enhanced by energy. If you doubt this, before your next sexual encounter try some dancing or other moderate exercise that energizes you. It can be very stimulating. As an interesting aside, ethologists observe that animals often chase each other around before a sexual encounter, and this energizing behavior could be one biological function of such behavior. While sexual arousal is associated with energy, there can be varying degrees of tension present, depending on the degree of inhibition or anxiety. However, if tension increases too much, sexual dysfunction is likely to be the result. Tense energy may be sexually invigorating, but if the tension is raised to such a high degree that you are experiencing a relative state of tense tired-ness, sexual dysfunction can be expected.

One of the important reasons that I see sexual arousal as underlaid by energy is the biological significance of such an association. Like anger, sexual behavior calls for high energy. Both of these emotions are very basic—one is critical for procreation and the other for fending off oppo-nents and aggressors. Such biological conditions demand high energy, and in the case of unrestrained activity, low tension. But tension may play a role with anger and sexual behavior if an individual inhibits himself because of circumstances.

What Is the Function of Moods?

Why do we even have moods? To answer this question, we must first understand that moods are biopsychological phenomena. They are not just something in our heads; rather, they have definite biological under-pinnings. Since that is the case, it follows that moods must perform an important function for us, because virtually every system of the body has evolved to have some adaptive value for survival and propagation of our species or it would have dropped out, or become vestigial, in the continu-ous culling that occurs in the evolutionary process.

So, what is the function of our moods? I believe that moods represent a kind of signal system. They give us vital information about our momen-tary condition, and if we utilize the information properly it enables us to maintain our bodies in peak physical condition and to meet in the most optimal way the inevitable stresses that afflict us. Millions of years of nat-ural selection have guaranteed that our moods have an adaptive value.[24] What we must do is discover that value and use it to our immediate advantage. I am convinced that proper awareness, understanding, and uti-lization of our moods can enable us to avoid maladaptive behaviors as well as to lead productive and happy lives.

Energy

At their most basic function, energetic moods signal or inform us of resources, and we can make decisions based on that knowledge.[25] When we become aware of these moods we can take action, and even when we are only vaguely aware of our moods, they may still motivate us. Utilizing and sharpening awareness of our moods confer a considerable advantage. For example, we can plan activities based on naturally occurring energy variations. (We shall see in the next chapter that we now know a lot about how to predict energy variations.)

Energetic moods especially motivate physical activity. If you are feeling very energetic, it is unpleasant to sit and do nothing. When you have lots of energy, intense mental activity may suffice, but physical activity is best. If you doubt this, start paying attention to your energy levels. For a few days, notice when they are high, moderate, and low, and the next time you have a burst of high energy, think about what activity is most appealing. You will see that sitting in a chair and relaxing is not appealing. Energy motivates you to *do* something. If you are resolved to exercise more, you are most likely to carry out this plan if you can begin your exercise during a high-energy period. This may be the key to being able to maintain an exercise program.

Since physical activity is most appealing in your highest energy periods, you may find that sedentary mental activity is slightly less appealing. But moderately high energy seems best for mental activity. Thus, it may be best to schedule sedentary work requiring lots of concentration in periods when you are feeling energetic but probably not at your highest energy. Nevertheless, given the well-established principle of individual differences, observing yourself to learn how *you* react is the wisest course. Once determined, the relationship between energy and mental activity will probably be a reliable pattern. [26]

Energetic moods also bolster us against adversity. The most difficult situation is made easier when you feel very energetic. Energetic moods represent what is common in such feelings as strength, power, hardiness, potency, stamina, endurance, vitality, and fortitude, just to mention a few. These are important signals about our current state, and they inform us when to start projects and when to persevere. Once again, knowing when your naturally high-energy periods are likely to occur allows you an advantage in being able to schedule your most stressful activities when your energy is high. This is a very important principle.

Low-energy or tiredness also informs us of something important, in this case, of reduced resources. The message of low-energy feelings is to rest and recuperate. Low energy moods represent signals from your body that you have done enough and that now you must have time for rejuvenation. Another vital way that low-energy moods influence us is in relation to food. When energy drops and we cannot immediately rest, we seek alternative energy sources—often food. Using this information wisely can enable you to avoid maladaptive behaviors. Stressful activities, for example, can be rescheduled during times of greater resources. Like feelings of high energy, moods indicating low energy represent vital information and, if utilized properly, give us considerable adaptive advantage.

Avoiding activity when we experience a low-energy mood may seem automatic and without any particular decision involved, but this is probably because the decision-making is habitual and occurs almost instantaneously. Thus, when we think about doing something and we notice that we are tired, we may not say to ourselves, "I'm tired, and I'd better not do that," but information about our current energy level is likely to contribute to our decision. By becoming more aware in these ways you begin to realize why maladaptive behaviors occur and how they can be forestalled. For example, you may give up an exercise plan that you vowed you never would abandon because you didn't exercise when you were exhausted one evening. Maybe breaking your resolve made you feel like a failure and caused you to give up. But being able to predict low-energy times or taking account of temporary low-energy periods enables you to continue the exercise program in an intelligent way during your next high-energy time.

Just as energy bolsters us against adversity, so low-energy moods make us vulnerable to adversity. Thus, anxiety can be magnified if energy is low. When your energy is high, an activity may be pleasurable and there is an absence of stress, but when you are tired the same activity can induce tension and be stressful. This information is very useful to know, and as a rule, whenever you feel stressed you should immediately notice your energy level. If you are tired and have little energy, stress can be expected even with activities that otherwise do not cause stress. This extends beyond stressful activities to the ways you think about yourself and your problems. When your energy is low, your problems will loom much larger.

Tension

Tense moods signal potential danger. The danger may be only in our minds, or, more often than not, we may have little idea why we feel tense and anxious. (Incidentally, the classic distinction between *fear* and *anxiety* is that anxiety is a kind of fear in which you do not know what you are afraid of.) But when we are tense, anxious, or nervous, we sense that something is wrong, even if we don't know what it is. Caution occurs with tension. We are preparing for whatever may come, and its effect is most observable in tight muscles. There is a kind of pattern of restraint, in this case associated with muscle tension. You may notice when you are tense how the muscles of your back, neck, and face are tight—it is a kind of emergency action. You are in a holding pattern, so to speak. This is a kind of primordial bodily pattern that is best for maximal survival. In terms used in biological psychology, we would say that tension represents a "stop system," as opposed to energy, which is a "go system."

Just as our prehistoric ancestors on the plains at times were wary of predators and remained alert to the possibility of danger while quickly finishing their activities, so does the tense person stay vigilant in a general way and does not give undivided attention to the task at hand. You will notice this effect especially by seeing how difficult it is to remain focused on a particular task when you are tense. After all, it makes no sense to pay close attention to a report that you are working on when a saber-toothed tiger may pounce on you at any moment! Rather, when you are tense your attention is not focused unless it is on the danger itself; it is as though you are continuously scanning your environment for the problem, whatever it is. Partly for this reason, tense moods result in lower-quality work.

This absence of focused attention when you are tense reduces awareness of your body as well. Thus, the signals that your body regularly provides—perhaps about how much food is necessary for your immediate metabolic needs—may go unnoticed or be exaggerated in this tense state. Virtually every effective diet program advises you to pay attention to the signals that your body provides about what food you really need, but this kind of attention is difficult to sustain when you are tense. This is a particularly important deficit, because such information is essential for discriminating between hunger based on bodily deficits and appetites based on moods and emotions.

Because tension feels bad, we seek various ways of escaping from it—we self-regulate in whatever way makes us feel better. Food is an often-used remedy, of course. But other choices are better, such as exercise and methods like muscle relaxation and meditation that work well to reduce tension.

Calmness, or low tension, signals safety to us. In this state there is little danger. We can act without caution because at some level of awareness we have determined that we are safe from peril. Calmness indicates either little stress or that we have effectively dealt with otherwise stressful conditions. When we feel calm, we can fully attend to whatever is happening, including the information that our body is providing. In addition, we can be completely immersed in the situation at hand.

Calmness also builds confidence in a basic way that often is unrecognized. A good example of the confidence that is associated with calmness arises from analyses of self-efficacy, or the belief about how successful you will be at any particular task.[27] As I indicated earlier, psychotherapists pay a lot of attention to self-efficacy because often it is thought to be a necessary element in changing your behavior. Extensive research shows that beliefs about your ability to do something are the best predictors of success, and one of the essential indications of your belief is your awareness of how calm or tense you are during a stressful activity. For example, if you are giving a public speech, or just speaking up to your boss, and your voice chokes up because of anxiety, your self-efficacy is weakened and you will probably be less successful. But when you are calm while speaking, your self-efficacy is strengthened. Calmness provides an elemental confirmation that you can do it. Thus, your degree of tense arousal can build confidence or detract from it. Incidentally, research has shown that your self-efficacy can be raised with tension-reduction training, a kind of management of your mood.

The Effects of Energy and Tension on Eating and Exercise

From this analysis of the function of our most basic moods, you can see why moods associated with a mixture representing calm energy predispose us to move about in a relaxed kind of way, to exercise our bodies, and to experience the pleasure that this provides. Energy prompts natural physical activity, and the calmness assures us that there is not too much stress or time pressure for unhurried physical activity to occur. With calmness, our muscles are not tense, and they are ready for exercise.

Tense tiredness leads to a desire for food, a ready source of energy. As I suggested elsewhere, mood-generated appetites frequently arise because of a motive to seek energy based on an often unconscious sensing of needs in relation to immediate demands, to stress, or to a perceived emergency. This is likely to occur at such a low level of awareness as to leave little knowledge of causes, unless one carefully observes. Such appetites may be conceived of even more simply as learned adaptations—that is, learned ways of counteracting unpleasant moods by substituting them with a pleasant feeling. But even in this case, eating is based on an elemental sense of how to deal with the cause of the negative mood: more energy.

The many studies showing that depression, anxiety, boredom, and loneliness cause overeating make perfect sense because all those negative moods represent variations of tense tiredness. Food is one way of correcting this deficit, and we can see how food urges and appetites are tied to this kind of deficit. Once you recognize how tense tiredness motivates eating, you have an explanation for why maintaining a diet is so hard when your mood is negative. It also is clear why breaking a diet is likely to occur when energy is otherwise low—for example, in the afternoon or the evening.

We learn to self-regulate with food from the earliest age. Undoubtedly, there are differences in this respect, and some people self-regulate with food more than others, but all of us do this to some extent. Of course, exercise is an alternative to food, but it is slower, and depending on your learning history you may not even make the connection. Although the motivation to exercise is sapped by thoughts that exercise will be unpleasant, other thoughts of good-tasting foods entice us to immediate pleasure, not the delayed pleasure that the exercise provides.

Although tense tiredness is inconsistent with the desire for exercise, nevertheless, exercise can produce calm energy. To achieve that mood state, a certain amount of what I call "cognitive override" is necessary. Recognizing our avoidance of exercise because of the tense tiredness, and being aware that this mood can be changed by exercise, the solution is temporarily to override the negative mood. This may not be easy, but it can be done, often just by beginning slowly and relying on the energy generated by some movement to motivate further exercise. For example, plan only to walk to the corner instead of two miles and see what happens to your energy.

Depression is an example of a certain kind of tense tiredness that affects millions of people. When you are feeling depressed your resources are low, and this is represented in the absence of energy—a central symptom of depression. But there is also some tension present in depression.[28] It is not a state of calmness. The degree of tension may vary, of course, and we see some depressions—sometimes represented by the clinical term "agitated depression,"—that include a good deal of tension. But whether a lot or a little, there is usually some tension in depression. There also are a host of other thoughts associated with depression: sadness, hopelessness, low self-esteem. These thoughts are very consistent with tense tiredness, and the overall pattern of consistency between thoughts and moods is something that scientists have observed in numerous studies.

From this brief survey, it should be apparent that knowing the function of our moods is very important. It gives us the ability to predict mood effects that are undesirable. Thus, if you are under stress and feeling tense, you can predict when you will experience strong urges to eat unnecessarily by becoming aware of natural variations in energy. You also will be able to understand when and why exercise is appealing or very hard to accomplish. Once you recognize ways that you habitually self-regulate to change negative moods, you can choose alternative self-regulatory strategies instead. Exercise is one excellent alternative, but a basic understanding of energy and tension opens many alternative choices.

How a Little Tension, but Not Too Much, Can Raise Your Energy[29]

Mark, a twenty-year-old student in one of my classes, came to my office one day. It was near final examination time, and he was concerned about his grade. He was on academic probation because of low grades in other classes, and he did not do well in the first two examinations in my class. As we talked about how he might earn a passing semester grade, it became clear that he had not yet started preparing for the final examination, which was in two days. He hadn't even read much of the material on the reading list. He said he found the class very interesting, but when it came time to reading the assigned books and research articles he would feel tired, and usually he would find something else important to do instead. He admitted that this was a common pattern of his behavior, and he said that he just couldn't get motivated to study until a deadline was upon him.

Mark's procrastination is an example of how many people manage themselves. They procrastinate until they become so anxious about failure or other negative consequences that they are energized to get to work. What appears to happen here is that increasing tension from an impending deadline raises their energy, and with that they are able to work in a sustained and intensive way.

Mark's example and similar cases lead me to believe that the two kinds of mood influence each other. As tension (anxiety) increases from low to moderate levels, it seems to increase energy as well. From this we can see one way that tense energy occurs. Many people live their lives in this state, although tense energy doesn't always develop because of procrastination, as it did in Mark's case. Often it occurs because people take on too much work in too little time. This creates increasing tension, and this seems to energize them. Moreover, tense energy can lead to efficient work. But let's consider what happens when the tension isn't moderate but high.

Suppose that Mark was absent for a couple of meetings and he arrived at class one day only to discover that an examination was scheduled and that he had forgotten about it. Let's assume further that he was close to flunking out of college and that if he did poorly in this class, it would terminate financial support from his parents. Recognizing that he is totally unprepared for this important exam could raise his anxiety to very high levels. And rather than being energized, as he was when tense arousal increased to moderate levels, this kind of jolt could bring the opposite feeling—perhaps a low-level depression as tension rose to high levels. Instead of increased energy, he probably would feel decreased energy. In this kind of situation, tense tiredness occurs rather than tense energy. Low energy coupled with high tension is a common pattern.

The fact that high tension and low energy often are coupled has another important implication. In my view, when our energy drops we become much more vulnerable to tension-inducing stress. This means that when our energy is low, all kinds of things bother us more than they otherwise would. You may have noticed that when you are tired, you are more irritable and you feel like snapping at people in ways that might be unusual for you. Parents are especially aware of the times when their little children are crabby and troublesome to deal with; it occurs when the children are tired. Low energy makes us more susceptible to anxiety and tension. That is why I say that stress has a greater impact during periods of tense tiredness. And as we have seen already, low energy and tiredness drive us to seek immediate remedies for this unpleasant state. The most common method of self-regulation, of course, is an energy-dense food—sugar, for example. The next time you have an urge for the kind of food that you don't need, I think you will find you are in a condition of tense tiredness.

Now we can see the picture of the complex relationship between energetic and tense arousal (see Figure 6.2). I believe that tension raises energy, but only up to a point. Beyond that, increasing tension reduces energy. And with reduced energy we become more vulnerable to stress with the result of even more tension—and often more sugar snacking.

The point at which increasing tension is no longer associated with increased energy—the point at which energy drops—depends on such things as your overall physical condition. For example, if Mark had been burning the candle at both ends, sleeping very little, and eating poorly, a relatively small amount of tension could be expected to reduce his energy. In other words, if he were in poor physical condition, even moderate demands would result in tense tiredness rather than tense energy. Here is where he could expect a sugar jag.

FIGURE 6.2

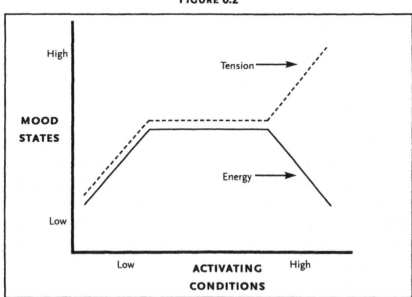

Now think about this, not in terms of the long-term physical condition of a person but in terms of changing energy levels at different times of day. If the unexpected examination occurred at Mark's high-energy time of day, it might result in tense energy, but if it were an otherwise low-energy time of day for him—say, late afternoon—then tense tiredness could be expected. And unhealthy methods of self-regulation could be expected.

Using this principle of how moderate levels of tension increase energy, but high tension reduces energy, you can see why the same activity can induce tension and stress at a low-energy time of day and little or no stress at a high-energy time of day. You also can see why an energy drain from loss of sleep or skipped meals often is associated with an unpleasant state of tense tiredness, and how correcting your energy deficit by taking a nap or eating a nutritious meal can shift your mood to the relatively more pleasant and productive condition of tense energy, or even to calm energy. It should also be clear why poor health leaves you much more vulnerable to increasing tension and the resultant tense tiredness, but exercising regularly and eating right raises your energy to the point where stress leaves you at least in a state of tense energy rather than tense-tiredness.

How Increasing Energy Can Elevate Tension, but Only Up to a Point

This same complex relationship occurs when *energy* is increasing. That is, increasing energy can raise tension to a point of tense energy, but high levels of energy seem to reduce tension to calm energy (Figure 6.3).

Daily energy cycles illustrate this phenomenon well. You may start out tired and calm in the morning, but as your energy increases, tension also rises, though perhaps not as rapidly. The tension is the result of stress, and while tension may be decreased in the low-energy time of sleep, the increasing energy of the day results in increased tension as well. But even though tense energy is a common condition for a person under stress, the highest energy of the day often is associated with calm energy. Moreover, energizing activities such as moderate exercise, eating, or even drinking coffee can leave you in a temporary state of calm energy. Calm energy also may occur if tension is reduced, so that tension-reducing activities

FIGURE 6.3

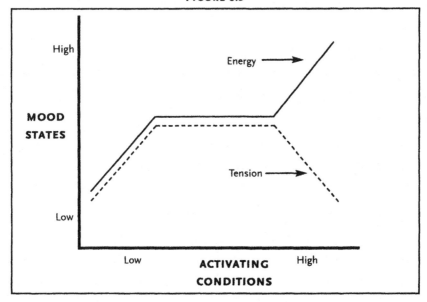

such as muscle relaxation, meditation, yoga, and massage produce calm energy. In all these examples in which energy rises above a certain point, calm energy is the result.

Exhaustion: Too Tired to Be Tense

Being aware of the changing patterns of energy and tension as bodily resources decline can be valuable for mood management. With stress at record levels, people often work to exhaustion, and this has important implications for eating and exercising. As an example, different ways of self-regulating mood, such as eating, tend to become more attractive in the initial stages of declining energy resources. But as one approaches exhaustion, the situation can be different. Also, feelings of exhaustion counteract well-meaning exercise programs, even though exercise may be the best way of managing stress.

To illustrate one aspect of exhaustion, recall that as resources decline, you feel less and less energy, and stress can increase. Tension is heightened, and tense tiredness becomes more apparent. Sleep-deprivation experiments demonstrate this shift clearly. Experimental subjects kept awake for two or three days first become irritable with lack of sleep. If you have ever stayed up all night, or even if you have just gotten too little sleep on several nights, you will experience the same increased irritability. As your energy drops, you gradually become tense and tired. But at some point the tension begins to decrease.

When sleep-deprived subjects were systematically observed in controlled research they first were irritable, but as sleep deprivation continued, their energy decreased to very low levels (increasing tiredness), and their irritability gradually was replaced with a kind of unreactive state.[30] In other words, when they were sufficiently tired, tension seemed to diminish or decline. They were exhausted. With exhaustion, tense tiredness shifts to a kind of calm tiredness.

The biological utility of reduced tension with exhaustion can be surmised fairly easily. Tense arousal is a warning system that keeps us alert to possible dangers. Among other things, this means staying awake—the sleeping animal is easy prey to the predator. Insomnia usually is caused by tension, and, at one level, this makes good biological sense. But eventually we need to sleep, or breakdown can be expected and, finally, death.[31] For recuperative rest and sleep to occur, tension (anxiety, fear) must be reduced. Therefore, as exhaustion develops, the tension diminishes.

To illustrate some points about body functioning, let's consider two kinds of exhaustion. First there is the exhaustion that occurs after a great deal of physical demand. This can drain your resources and leave your muscles unresponsive. But there is also a kind of exhaustion that comes from a high-stress lifestyle and too little sleep. This may not affect your musculature in the same way as intense physical exertion, but nonetheless you can feel used up or burned out. The two examples of exhaustion have different causes, but the mood reactions can be quite similar.

Backpackers and hikers will know what I am talking about by the exhaustion from a day of physically demanding hiking. At the end of one grueling hike, a companion of mine who had a mild snake phobia was totally unconcerned about snakes, although at the beginning of the hike she looked carefully where she was walking. Following a long hike, another hiker casually brushed insects off his food, unfazed when a few ended up being eaten—just a little more protein. These are examples of what happens when energy is drained and tense arousal is very low.

Substantial physical demand reduces energy to a very low level, and tension is reduced to such a degree that calm tiredness prevails. You become unresponsive to anything less than extreme tension-inducing circumstances. The dynamic interaction of energy and tension is especially clear with these experiences. This calm tiredness with exhaustion can be a very pleasant state. The usual concerns seem unimportant, unpleasant anxiety is eliminated, and rest or sleep is complete.

Exhaustion that occurs with stress and too little sleep can have a mood effect similar to heavy exercise at the end of a long day. If you have had the experience of doing too much and using needed sleep time to give yourself more waking hours, you will notice that at the end of the day you fall into bed exhausted. This part is pleasant, but before the time of exhaustion, and especially during the low-energy times of the day, tense tiredness is more likely to occur. And this is not a pleasant state.

The primary way we self-regulate our moods and feelings when we are exhausted is first to sleep, or at least rest. But with the tense tiredness that precedes exhaustion, other behaviors, especially eating, are much more likely. Exercise is not even an option because we feel too drained. These reactions are mainly true when stress and not physical exercise is the cause of declining resources.

We can see how declining resources and reduced energy lessen our desire to exercise and increase our urge to eat. But as exhaustion approaches, not only are physical movement and exercise avoided, but food temporarily may be of less interest. With exhaustion, however, basic replenishment of the body at some point becomes vital. One world-class marathon runner described how he slowly moves about in stony silence immediately after the run, unresponsive to anything. But then as he recovers a bit, he becomes voraciously hungry. The physically exhausted person is driven to replenish the system. In all these cases, however, moods are signals of need. Thus, understanding exhaustion and the stages that precede it can give us essential insight into the function and operation of mood states.

In the next three chapters we will focus on the many conditions under which energetic moods vary (for example, time of day, sleep, stress). And we will briefly survey the physiology that underlies our moods. We will also focus on how this information can be used intelligently to self-regulate moods. This information can yield valuable strategies for managing both your moods and the undesirable side effects of those moods, including overeating and avoiding exercise.

CHAPTER 7

Changes in Energy—and Mood

W HEN YOU START PAYING ATTENTION to your energy levels, you realize how much they change each day. Sometimes you feel energetic and sometimes you don't, but when your energy is high you feel good. You sense strength, confidence, optimism, and plea-sure; your mood is up. When your energy drops, however, everything looks different. Small tasks seem insurmountable and daily annoyances intolerable. When you think about energy this way, you can see what a powerful force it is.[1]

Manufacturers understand this, too, and they constantly bombard us with advertisements for ways to boost our energy levels: special kinds of foods, food supplements, vitamins, herbs, over-the-counter drugs, cof-fees, soft drinks. But the thoughtful person must question how many of these enticing products really work, and how much is simple sales pitch. The science of subjective energy is not developed to the point where there is certainty about these matters, but from a good deal of research we do know some basic principles about how energy feelings vary.

Because energy feelings are based on a complex and constantly chang-ing physiology, as well as on shifting events and circumstances, they rise and fall continuously. Moods inexorably follow daily cycles of energy as we mobilize ourselves, expend resources, replenish them, and become active again. The body is an energy system, and on any typical day we experience the greatest shifts in energy from sleep to wakefulness and, during the waking hours, from sedentary relaxation to vigorous physical activity. Food, thoughts, and emotions usually cause smaller shifts, unless the emotions are strong, in which case great changes in energy can occur.

Becoming aware of these shifts in energy can give us vital information about where our moods come from, why they change, and, ultimately, how we may be able to control them. Understanding our own energy rhythms is, in my view, one of the most significant prerequisites for managing our negative moods. It is one of the best ways of predicting when urges for unneeded food are likely to hit us—that is, when tension rises and energy declines. But most of us go through the day unaware of our energy patterns. If we get in the habit of monitoring our energy swings, patterns become easy to spot, and, once recognized, these insights can offer us a great deal of self-control.

One important reason for our lack of awareness is that our feelings of energy can be mixed with feelings of tension. Both tension and energy are activating, and many people do not separate the two kinds of feelings. Moreover, tension influences our energy levels, and it is less predictable than daily energy variations because tension can occur from momentary stressors, occasional thoughts about our problems, or other things. Thus, within the mixture of energy and tension that we experience each day, we tend to lose track of natural energy patterns.

Careful scientific research indicates that we typically experience a low point in energy on awakening, rising to a period of high energy in late morning or early afternoon. Then we usually lose energy in the late afternoon and evening. Often there is a lesser peak in energy in the early evening before a decline in the last part of the day. Within this daily energy pattern, shorter cycles of energy and tiredness occur periodically.[2] Thus, you may feel energetic at ten in the morning, experience a slight dip in energy at eleven, and another increase at noon, and these shorter cycles occur on top of our natural daily cycle. And there may be individual differences, so that so-called morning people reach their highest energy early in the day while so-called night people peak later in the day.[3]

Energy cycles are also affected by sleep periods, as evident in sleep-deprivation studies. My students sometimes "pull all-nighters," as they say, when they study throughout the night for an exam the next day. An interesting cycle of tiredness and energy usually occurs, and this illustrates the underlying *circadian* (twenty-four-hour) cycle. Students who are up all night will become increasingly tired until about midway through the normal sleep period, about 3:00 A.M., when they can hardly keep their eyes open. But from then on they become less tired, and by 7:30 or so the next morning, a normal waking time, they feel almost as alert as they would if they had slept all night—only to experience a crash later in the day.

The middle-of-the-night drop of energy to its lowest point indicates the time when self-regulation occurs in the form of extra food intake and consumption of caffeinated beverages for the person who must stay awake. This is an attempted energy boost. For the person who is feeling tense and can't sleep, a variety of drugs and other substances may be sought, including food, as a way to reduce tension in order to go to sleep. This low-energy period, when mixed with tension, can be a time when thoughts about personal problems may be very negative and can create even more tension.

Scientists study such biological rhythms extensively as part of a field called chronobiology or chronopsychology. In fact, virtually every biological function that has been observed over time shows cyclical variation: body temperature, heart rate, respiration, blood sugar, serotonin, and many more. Our moods are no exception; our energy cycles in particular show this rhythmic form. The patterns that are observed often are called *endogenous biological rhythms*, because they are largely influenced by bodily processes that are driven by a kind of biological clock.[4]

Besides the circadian rhythms already referred to, there is evidence of mood rhythms associated with so-called *infradian cycles* (longer than twenty-four hours), such as the female menstrual cycle, seasonal rhythms as in Seasonal Affective Disorder (SAD), and even lifelong cycles of energy from youth to old age.[5]

The endogenous nature of our energy rhythms, and how they make us feel more or less alert and energetic, becomes obvious when we fly across time zones. Flying from New York to Europe, for example, results in disruptions of these rhythms that we refer to as jet lag. Our internal rhythms are disrupted because we are now encountering hours of light, darkness, sleeping, waking, eating, and physical activity that are very different from those our body is used to. Essentially when traveling this way, we join a new time culture, and this disrupts many basic biological rhythms.

Energy Rhythms and Tension Changes

In one recent study that I conducted, thirty-one males and females between eighteen and fifty-five years of age systematically rated their energy and tension levels with an adjective checklist every hour of the day, from the time they awakened in the morning until they went to sleep at night. They followed this procedure during three typical days in a period of several weeks. Rating their mood took only a few seconds, but the average person made these ratings sixteen or seventeen times a day for three days, so it was a demanding task. Many of the participants remembered to make their ratings by wearing watches that beeped every hour.

The energy cycle that was evident in this study had the same pattern as that observed in other studies that my students and I had previously conducted. The average waking time for this group was 7:45 A.M., and at that time these participants rated their energy level as one of the lowest points of the day. But their energy level rose sharply in the first hours of the morning, and reached its highest point at noon. After 1:00, energy began a decline that lasted throughout the afternoon and, following another small peak at 7:00 in the evening, it further declined to the lowest point of the day, which for this group averaged 11:28 P.M. The peaks and troughs observed in this study are consistent with other studies, but they vary somewhat depending on the sample of people who are self-rating.

These participants not only rated their energy hourly but also their tension. Thus, the two central elements of mood—energy and tension—were obtained every hour for three days, and, therefore, it was possible to observe the natural circadian energy cycle and its interaction with tension. Figure 7.1 shows the pattern that occurred.

For this group, tension was also the lowest of the day upon waking. This is common for most people, but if an individual is experiencing serious depression a different pattern may be observed.[6] For this group of healthy volunteers, tension increased throughout the first part of the day, with the negative state reaching its peak at about 5:00 P.M. and declining somewhat in the last part of the day. In this study people were experiencing stress as part of a normal daily pattern, and, therefore, some tension could be expected. If they had been on vacation for a couple of weeks—it takes about a week of vacation to relax—they may have experienced relatively little tension throughout the day.

FIGURE 7.1

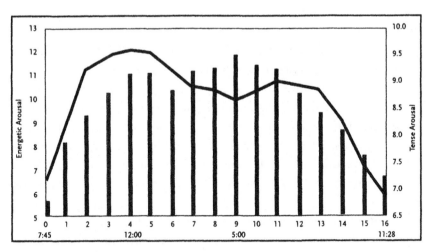

Energetic arousal (line) and tense arousal (bar) as a function of time of day

The relationship between energy and tension is critical for understanding our everyday behavior and especially our tendencies to exercise and to eat. When our energy is high, we can withstand stress with relative impunity. But as our energy drops, we become much more vulnerable to anxiety or tension. As a consequence, stress can have its greatest effect when energy is low. As I said before, the same activity can produce little stress during a period of high energy, but in low-energy times that activity can raise tension and increase stress. One negative effect of this period of tense tiredness is that we often do things we would prefer not to do to self-regulate the unpleasant state, including eating.

Looking at the results of this study of healthy men and women, we can see that the morning and early afternoon, between 10:00 A.M. and 1:00 P.M., represented a time of high energy and relatively low tension. Even though they experienced the normal daily stresses we all do, we can assume that during this period of relative calm energy, the stressors in their lives had less impact. But in the period between 3:00 and 7:00 P.M., their energy and tension shifted. During this time, tense tiredness was much more evident, and a similar kind of tense tiredness occurred in the last two hours of the day.

Many of the students who volunteered for this study were psychology majors, so it may be safe to assume they were fairly self-aware. My experience with such students is that they exercise regularly and take reasonably good care of their health. Even so, however, this group experienced periods of tense tiredness, when less healthy behaviors could be expected. If we were to conduct this same study with people who do not take care of themselves well, and who are under more stress, energy would probably be lower and tension higher throughout the day. We could expect relatively little time of calm energy for them each day and more tense tiredness. Of course, for this less healthy group the times of day when the typical person experiences peaks in energy—late morning or early afternoon, and early evening—probably would be only marginally better.

The declining energy that occurs at various times each day, and the increased vulnerability to stress-produced tension, leaves most people subject to undesirable and sometimes urgent methods of self-regulation. Although more optimal ways of counteracting the tense tiredness such as moderate exercise may be employed, many people succumb instead to the most expedient means: food. Everyone is affected this way, but in my view people with so-called eating disorders are likely to be even more affected by circadian energy changes. In the next section we will discuss a behavior pattern that is not technically classified as an eating disorder, but that many people feel borders on such a classification.

Night-Eating Syndrome

Overeating as a way of seeking energy and feeling better when faced with unpleasant anxiety or tension is most likely to occur when resources drop—for example, late in the afternoon or at night. One pattern of this type of overeating, first observed in the 1950s by Albert Stunkard, has been the subject of numerous scientific papers.[7] Called night-eating syndrome, it is not currently classified in DSM-IV as an eating disorder, but it is associated with obesity and parallels the energy and tension cycle we are examining. People with night-eating syndrome eat as much as half or more of their daily food intake at night. They often experience insomnia, poor sleep, and frequent awakenings, during which they consume large amounts of food. In the morning, on the other hand, they usually eat relatively little. Several researchers have identified stress and evening tension as influences on night-eating syndrome.[8] People with this syndrome tend to be obese, which is not surprising because of the metabolic consequences of their habit: little energy expenditure through physical activity, but a great deal of energy intake from the food. One researcher described personal interviews with obese night eaters who said they felt distressed and hopeless by their inability to stop eating at night, although they could maintain their diet during the day.[9]

Notice the similarity between the conditions observed among night eaters and many other people with less severe symptoms of overeating. For example, night eaters overeat during periods of low energy—nighttime. They awaken frequently and have other kinds of troubled sleep patterns, indicating the strong possibility that they are experiencing heightened tension. Sleep problems often are caused by tension or anxiety, and when this condition is reduced, more normal sleeping occurs. Similarly, when sleep problems are reduced among those with night-eating syndrome, the eating problems can abate.

With night-eating syndrome, then, the overeating occurs during a period of low energy and increased tension. This tense tiredness is exactly the condition that motivates many people to eat. Moreover, the experience of night eaters of feeling distressed and hopeless is quite understandable because this tense-tired time leads to negative perceptions of yourself and your future. Furthermore, the low energy present at night makes it more difficult to resist the temptations of good-tasting food. Using a term that diet researchers often employ, the low energy that people experience results in *disinhibition*. The usual levels of inhibition against overeating probably are dependent on energy, so in low-energy periods we are vulnerable to the temptations of food.

Self-Observation of Energy and Tension

Knowing your daily patterns of energy and tension can enable you not only to predict when the best periods of the day are likely to occur (calm energy) but to anticipate times of tense tiredness, when unwanted urges and other maladaptive behaviors may emerge. This allows you to understand why you react the way you do, and possibly to plan counteractive measures. For example, if you observe your energy cycle and the times when stress and tension usually occur, you could arrange timely exercise sessions to help counteract food urges that often occur during tense tired periods. You also will know when exercise probably will be most attractive, and this is of no small benefit if you have difficulty staying with an exercise program. You may also want to schedule your most challenging work of the day when your energy is high and your tension is low, thus allowing you to be most productive.

In one of the classes that I teach, students regularly complete this kind of self-study, and it has become a favorite activity. It is time-consuming and a bit difficult, but it pays great dividends. Not only is this information useful for understanding eating and exercise, but a number of my students have told me that they use it to plan the times that they will study or relax. They also learn when their personal problems will seem magnified, and try to avoid thinking about them then.

If you decide to do this kind of self-study, you should do it over a period of three days. These days should be typical for you. You should get up and go to bed at about the same time and do the same kinds of activities. Since your object will be to identify your body's natural energy cycle, these days should involve patterns of waking, sleeping, and activity that occur on most days. Establish a fixed procedure when you will rate yourself—for example, at the top of every hour, from waking in the morning until bedtime. Use a seven-point scale, from the most energy experienced each day to the least. Next, you can graph the average energy and tension ratings at each hour (use different color pencils). Then connect the energy points throughout the day and draw bars for tension levels (refer back to Figure 7.1).

When you have finished, look carefully at the hours of the day when you usually have the highest energy and lowest tension. These will be indications of the times you usually experience calm energy. Then look at the hours when your tension is highest and energy is lowest. These tense-tired times are likely to be when unwanted food urges occur, as well as other psychological problems.

As you become more adept at identifying your energy and tension levels, you might continue this self-study by observing yourself even more carefully at certain times of day. For example, suppose you notice that you are especially tempted to break your diet in the late afternoon, as is common. You probably will find that before breaking your diet, your energy has begun to flag and you are feeling a bit tired. You may also notice that you are a little less patient than you have been. Other indications of tension may be that things are bothering you more than they usually do. Thoughts of good-tasting foods may come into your head, and a food urge may threaten to overwhelm your dietary resolve. One of my students who was a particularly good self-observer told a class on mood that whenever she thought about ice cream and suddenly wanted some, she knew she was slightly tense and tired. Being able to determine when you have slipped from a calm-energetic mood into tense tiredness will be extremely valuable to you.

Moreover, it is profitable to observe the gradual drop in your energy level and increasing tension *while it is occurring*. I have found it easier to prevent excessive tense tiredness if I can catch it before it takes over. Then I try to do something to raise my energy, reduce tension, or both. This can be something as simple as a short brisk walk. If I have skipped a meal, and lack of food is contributing to the drop in energy, a small nutritious snack gives me a little boost. If lack of sleep is the problem, a short nap may do the trick. A few minutes of a stress-management exercise can often be helpful, too. This might involve muscle relaxation, visualization, or meditation. Through practice, you can figure out what works best for you.

Tense Tiredness and Negative Thoughts

Sometimes you don't notice that your mood has changed for the worse. If you were feeling energetic and now you are slightly tense, you may not notice it immediately. But when you start observing yourself carefully, you will realize that there are other indications of this negative mood state. For example, as your mood declines, your thoughts gradually become more negative. This does not always happen, but it has been observed often enough in careful scientific research that a term has been coined to describe this association between moods and thoughts. It is called *mood congruence*, and it is simply the tendency of our thoughts to match a positive or negative mood.[10]

An example of mood congruence is the tendency of depressed people to remember and dwell on only the negative things that have happened to them. If you talk to a depressed friend, you will notice that only the bad features of life seem to be in focus. You may find yourself advising this friend to concentrate instead on the positive aspects of his or her life, and your friend may try, but the negative thoughts will keep intruding.

This match between our moods and thoughts occurs because the body works as an integrated whole. In other words, the many systems of the body are not independent but interrelated. Thus the cognitive and mood systems are interdependent, and each influences the other. You can see this in the way that some cognitive theories of depression rely on changing your thoughts as a way of influencing your moods. But the association works the other way as well, so that your moods can influence your thoughts, and it is this kind of influence that I wish to talk about next.

I started thinking about this some years ago when I had been observing circadian energy rhythms and noticing the natural pattern that occurs day after day. The more I observed this energy cycle, the more I became convinced of the way it influences many aspects of behavior. At that time I was troubled by a personal problem, and I noticed that I would tend to think about it and be bothered by it while trying to go to sleep at night. I would get to sleep, however, and some time the next morning the problem would come to mind again. It was striking to me that in the morning it did not appear nearly as serious. The same problem seemed more serious at night than it did the next morning. Why?

It seemed to me that, apart from the troubling issue itself, this changing perception of how serious the problem appeared might represent a significant psychological process. When I mentioned it to my students and colleagues, without exception they all said that the same thing had happened to them. The more I observed it, the more certain I became that the phenomenon was related to my circadian energy rhythm. At night, when my energy was low and I felt tense, the problem appeared serious, even unsolvable; in the morning, when my energy was increasing, the problem appeared less serious. It had to be understood in relation to my mood.

Changing Perceptions of Our Problems

I decided to study this phenomenon and recruited a group of volunteers who had an unremitting personal problem, the kind that continues day after day.[11] One woman was experiencing a painful marital separation, another had unyielding weight problems that bothered her continually, and a third had problems with severe parental discord.

Each participant met with me to establish what the problem was, and then he or she was given a packet of rating scales to carry around to rate the seriousness of the problem at different times. On ten separate days, five times a day, these volunteers would think about the problem for a short while, then rate how serious it appeared to them and how likely it was that it might be solved. They were carefully instructed to evaluate the problem only at that moment and not to consider previous ratings. They also rated their energy and tension at those times.

Four of the five times each day represented different points on the circadian energy cycle: just after awakening, in the late morning or early afternoon, in the late afternoon, and just before they intended to go to sleep. They also did their ratings one other time each day, just after they had taken a brisk ten-minute walk. This could be any time of day, but it had to be at least two hours earlier or later than any other rating, and the same time on all ten days. From the many ratings that were done each day I was able to determine how serious the problem appeared to these people when their energy was either naturally high or low.

The results of this experiment clearly indicate that time of day subtly influences our perception of personal problems. On any given day, the problem sometimes seemed more serious, sometimes less, but when the ratings were combined, most participants rated the problem as more serious and less likely to be solved in the late afternoon than in the late morning. Although this difference was small, it was statistically significant. The problem also was rated as more serious late at night and in the early morning than at mid-morning, but these differences did not reach statistical significance.

Not everyone had the same times of day of high and low periods of energy and tension, so in another analysis I compared problem perception at whatever time the individual indicated was his or her highest energy and lowest tension. The result? Irrespective of time of day, the problem appeared most serious whenever people felt least energetic and most tense.

Figure 7.2 on the next page shows these differences. Without considering the brisk walk for a moment, notice how the average energy level (light gray bar) is low on waking and reaches its highest point at late morning but then drops off at late afternoon and before sleep. Tension (dark gray bar) did not vary a great deal during the day for this group, but

FIGURE 7.2

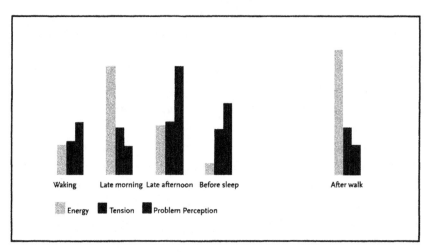

Waking   Late morning Late afternoon Before sleep   After walk

Energy   Tension   Problem Perception

Energy, tension, and perception of personal problems

it was highest in the late afternoon. These results parallel those in Figure 7.1. The personal problem was rated as most serious (black bar) at late afternoon and next most serious before sleep.

The problem ratings after the ten-minute brisk walk, although it occurred at different times of day, were considerably diminished as the energy of the participants was raised. The energy was even higher after the walk than it was at late morning, the highest natural energy level of the day. (It did not reduce tension dramatically, however.) This and other studies generally show that following a walk, you will feel about as much energy as you would at the highest energy period of the day.[12]

The energizing effects of moderate exercise can affect the way you evaluate your problems. The next time you are worrying about a personal problem, especially if you feel tense and tired, go for a brisk ten-minute walk, and notice how the problem appears to you afterward.

Can We Think Ourselves into a Good Mood?

I am often asked whether it is possible for us to control our moods by regulating our thoughts, and the answer I give is a qualified yes. It certainly is possible theoretically. As I said previously, the many systems of our body are fully integrated and they operate in a holistic fashion. The head doesn't act without bodily concurrence, so to speak, and vice versa. The often-observed mood congruence that I described (negative moods correlated with negative thoughts) is a good example of this, and congruence suggests not only that moods can influence thoughts but that thoughts can influence moods. But accomplishing this kind of mood control by the right thinking is not easy. Especially in the throes of an intense mood—depression, for example—we find it almost impossible to "snap out of it" by changing our thoughts. But there is a broad array of positive findings on cognitive control of moods, and cognitive therapies of depression enjoy wide support.[13]

My own research certainly shows that most people resort to cognitive self-regulation of bad moods—in other words, they try to change their thinking.[14] Controlling thoughts was one of the most popular strategies among people in one broad survey. When adults are faced with a bad mood, over half of them attempt to think positively, or they concentrate on something else, trying not to let it bother them. They may also try to give themselves a pep talk. Such cognitive techniques are among the most successful ways of changing mood.

One individual difference we found in our research about how people change a bad mood is that men tend to use these cognitive practices more often than women do. But the way this is done isn't obvious, as is evident from the fact that men may be more successful in controlling depression by *avoiding* thinking about their problems, especially ruminative thinking. Some scientists such as Susan Nolen-Hoeksema at the University of Michigan believe that the tendency to ruminate about a problem is one reason women are twice as likely as men to be depressed.[15] Thus, while women may continue to think about a problem until it is overwhelming, men use hobbies or other ways of distracting themselves from that kind of thinking.

Men are not always more successful than women at dealing with depression and other negative moods, however. In our research we found that, compared to men, professional women tend to use the best ways of changing a bad mood, including thought control. Men are significantly more likely to use drugs and alcohol to control their negative moods than are women. Women may be twice as likely as men to be depressed, but men are three times as likely as women to be alcoholics—and alcohol is probably used at least in part as a way of self-medicating against negative moods.[16]

Energy Variations in Sickness and Health

Al works out at the same health club where I do. He is seventy years old, but most people would guess he is in his fifties. Al is well liked by everyone. Usually he is filled with energy and there is calmness about him that is distinctive. (Incidentally, he is not a bit overweight.) Ordinarily he is extremely sociable, but one day I saw him working out alone on an exercise bicycle, and when I asked how he was doing, he said, "Not so good. I have had a heavy cold for two days, and it has sapped my energy. I was laying around the house, and then I realized that without my usual exercise, I feel more drained, so I decided to come today and do a light workout." The fact that Al was not socializing with one of his friends was unusual, but it demonstrated his lack of energy.[17] The depleted energy that Al felt from the cold is a very common effect of illness.[18] When a systemic illness strikes, we often want to go to bed because we don't have the energy for anything else.

Nowhere is the close association between mood and the body more evident than when we are sick. Physicians are well aware that the "chief complaint" of most general medical patients is tiredness or lack of energy. This was apparent, for example, in one study of 500 medical patients seen in a general medical facility in the Boston area.[19] Thirty-seven percent said they had been very tired, often for months, before seeking treatment. A good case can be made that an energy drop is like an early-warning system for general illness.

The relationship of energy level to both physical and psychological illness was especially apparent in a study of highly educated nurses (master's degree) carried out by Jane Dixon and her colleagues at Yale University.[20] The 310 nurses did extensive self-assessments of their health at present and in previous decades. Because of their training and experience, they could be expected to have a very accurate view of these conditions. Energy level emerged as the best predictor of both physical and psychological health: when they were more healthy their energy was high, and sickness was associated with lack of energy. Mood is more than just a disembodied feeling; it is a good measure of the state of your whole being.

The relationship between mood and illness has been strikingly demonstrated in studies of susceptibility to the common cold. One study involved 394 otherwise healthy subjects who volunteered to go to a special medical facility and have rhinoviruses or a placebo dripped directly into their noses. Medical examination then determined who contracted colds and who did not.[21] The good news is that only 38 percent of those who received the actual virus got colds. One of the best predictors of who would become ill was mood. If the present and past moods of these people were bad, they were more likely to contract the cold. So, the next time you are sitting next to someone who is sneezing and blowing his nose, don't be so certain you will catch his cold, because even if his germs are deposited directly into your nose, you probably won't succumb. But if your mood is bad and has been negative in recent days, you should beware.

Another common malady related to mood is headache. It is estimated that up to one-third of adults suffer from bouts of headache, and mood is a good predictor of when headaches will occur. In one recent study of episodic tension-type headaches in which sufferers rated their moods over fourteen consecutive days, levels of tense arousal were significant predictors of headache occurrence.[22] In other words, those who often experienced headaches were significantly more tense than control subjects, even when they weren't having headaches. Moreover, for headache sufferers, the actual headache involved significant tension and fatigue.

Mood is related to health in another important way. Infectious diseases are warded off or contracted by changes in our immune system, and this system varies all the time—as do our moods.[23] Moreover, as remarkable as it may seem, you can predict when your immune system will be functioning best by judging your mood. This has been demonstrated in a number of well-controlled studies. In one study by researchers at the State University of New York, medical students rated their mood over eight weeks at the same time as their immune system functioning was assessed.[24] Ratings of mood on each day of testing showed that the immune-system response was lower on days of negative mood and higher on days of positive mood. More recently, a study of natural killer cell activity showed that this measure of immune system function was predicted by positive and negative moods.[25] If you think about this when your mood is up, you can almost envision the killer cells circulating through your bloodstream and vanquishing sickness-producing invaders.

The close association between the immune system and mood also may be understood with reference to sleep—one of the most important influences on energy level. For example, some research shows that even a modest loss of sleep reduces your body's immune response.[26] In the next section we look at the vital association between sleep and energy level.

The Value of Sleep

Americans sleep fewer hours today than a decade ago. The tremendous toll in accidents and work loss is obvious, but another immediate effect of this sleep starvation is negative mood. You can understand why this occurs because energy and mood are so closely related, and sleep is one of the most important influences on energy. Two recent books by well-known sleep scientists William Dement from Stanford University and James Maas from Cornell University agree completely on how sleep loss results in deteriorated mood.[27] Reviewing sleep-deprivation studies, Dement says, "The effect of sleep deprivation on mood in the average healthy person is potentially a huge, invisible problem. Sleep-deprivation studies have shown consistently that sleep-deprived subjects are more irritable, more volatile, and more depressed than control subjects."[28]

In one careful investigation by David Dingus and his colleagues at the University of Pennsylvania, healthy young adults were studied over the course of seven consecutive nights in which they were allowed to sleep only four to five hours each night—33 percent less sleep than they usually got.[29] This shortened sleep pattern is not unlike what many stress-plagued people experience all the time. Dingus found clear and solid evidence of cumulative effects of this deprivation: fatigue (low energy), tension, confusion, mental exhaustion, and stress. This cumulative sleep debt had an escalating effect on daytime sleepiness, and recovery from the seven nights of partial sleep loss required two nights of full sleep. Dingus's findings are reflected in other studies as well.[30]

How much sleep do we actually need? A few years ago, the National Commission on Sleep Disorder Research, made up of many of the best sleep scientists in the world, concluded that Americans are severely sleep-deprived and, therefore, dangerously sleepy during the day.[31] They went on to say that the vast majority of adults need a nightly average of at least seven hours of sleep to avoid the consequences of sleep deprivation, and many individuals require more than eight hours. But the average person is sleeping fewer than seven hours a night.[32] In effect, what this shows is that the average person usually experiences sleep deprivation, with all the negative mood effects that this implies.

In a class that I teach, students keep a stress journal over a number of weeks, recording their daily mood levels as well as the influence of variables such as the previous night's sleep. These journals consistently show not only that sleep loss affects mood (and thus energy and tension), but also that a variety of other negative effects subsequently emerge that are associated with increased stress levels. The effects of sleep loss are subtle, but ultimately very significant.

Although the relationship between sleep and mood is evident once you begin to observe yourself carefully, many people (perhaps most) are unaware of the effects of their sleep deficit—even though their mood may be bad, and they may be self-regulating by overeating, and even though the sleep loss may be sabotaging their exercise plans.

Many people have surprisingly come to regard sleep as expendable, as an activity that can be shortened with few consequences. I am reminded of a recent talk, during which a member of the audience, a young man, asked, "Can you give us any information on how to sleep less? I don't like wasting time sleeping. I want to be like Thomas Edison who slept hardly at all." He was voicing an opinion that lots of people have about the unimportance of sleep. People with full agendas often don't realize that more rather than less sleep will keep their mood up. I told the young man that Edison is reputed to have taken frequent and long naps and that if this young man were looking for models of superior functioning, he might consider Albert Einstein, who felt he needed ten hours of sleep to do his best work.

Taking naps to regenerate energy should be commonly practiced by many sleep-starved people today. Indeed, in many parts of the world the siesta has been a fine tradition. One of the most enjoyable and productive conferences I ever attended took place in Spain. Papers were given and lively discussions followed, filling up our mornings and evenings, but in the afternoons we had a good meal followed by a nap or some other form of recreation.[33] Few Americans turn to this method to feel more energetic.

When people who need more sleep tell me why they don't nap, they usually say it is because napping disrupts their energy and makes them feel groggy afterward. I suspect that they are sleeping too long or at the wrong time of day (fifteen to thirty minutes in the afternoon is best). Or they may be unaware that they need to allow time to recover their energy following a nap. Awakening from a nap is something like awakening in the morning: unless there is an emergency, you don't jump up fully awake. A bit of experimentation with napping can yield great benefits. [34]

Are Your Moods Caused by Things That Happen to You?

Stress from daily life leads to tension, a state we have seen often results in decreased energy and a bad mood. This, in turn, can lead to overeating and avoidance of exercise. As greater demands are placed on us than we can cope with, our resources become drained and tension grows. But cognition—our mental state—can play an important part in this process of escalating tension and declining mood.

When we become tense because of negative things that happen to us in the course of daily life, the tension usually is based on our interpretations, expectations, or other cognitive reactions. Being late for an appointment or having too much to do can be stressful, primarily because we *perceive* it as negative. If somehow we could change our interpretation of the significance of being late—in other words, if we could see things differently—we could have an immediate impact on our own stress level. [35] This is why cognitive theories of stress management place a great deal of emphasis on cognitively reconstructing a situation so that it appears less threatening. The value of this approach is supported by much scientific research, and it is certainly something I recommend. [36]

Personal problems certainly contribute to our overall stress level. If something is bothering us, each time we think of it we can become tense. This can go on over a long period. Continuing personal problems can lead to chronic high tension, with all its associated physical troubles and dysfunctional behaviors. Cognitive processes are important here as well. Something is a problem for us because we interpret it that way, and if somehow we could change our interpretation, it would be less of a problem.

This matter of interpretation brings up complicated issues of unconscious influences. We may not always be fully aware of the troubling things in our lives but they still bother us. There are different points of view about these so-called unconscious influences. Many cognitive scientists prefer to talk about low levels of awareness, to differentiate this from a Freudian-like dynamic unconscious. But most researchers agree that we aren't aware about a good deal of cognitive activity that still affects us, or at least our conscious awareness is very low. Nonetheless, whether we are fully aware of the problem or not, the effect of it is usually increased tension. And, as we have seen in the last chapter, this often results in lower energy as well. From these matters we can see that our problems influence our moods.

Our energy level is also of vital importance to how we react, as well as to our thoughts and interpretations of events. Most of us try to find a reason for our bad moods: "Something happened to me, and it gave me a bad mood." Sometimes this is the case, but we also must think about naturally occurring bodily processes—including health, sleep, food, and physical activity—that are often more important causes of our overall mood than events that occur in our life.

To say this differently, a feeling of increased tension based on how we look at the situation is likely to be the main way that moods are affected by stress, negative events, or personal problems. If our energy is high, however, the elevated tension will have a relatively benign mood effect. You may have noticed sometimes in the past that even though bad things were happening, your mood remained positive. But it is clear that if our energy is depleted, increasing tension brought on by stressful events or by thinking about a problem can worsen an already bad mood. In fact, if your energy is low enough, even minor problems or stress can have a devastating effect, and often they can drive you to self-regulate by eating or other unwanted behaviors.

Similarly, with good moods, natural processes that elevate energy are likely to be the main reason you feel good. This is not to say that if you learn you just won the lottery, you wouldn't be in a good mood for a while. You undoubtedly would. Positive events can energize you, even a simple thing like a compliment. And certainly looking forward to something positive can raise your mood.[37] But in my experience these passing influences are less important to our good moods than natural processes that raise our energy level: good health, quality sleep, proper nutrition, plenty of enjoyable exercise, and maintenance of good physical condition in general.

When you understand your moods in these ways, you can see why they often seem mysterious—as though they come and go without reason. If things that happen to you were the main causes of your moods, you would soon be perfectly aware of the reasons for your good and bad moods. But that isn't the case. Most people are puzzled by their moods. This is because the natural processes that influence our moods change slowly, and the shifts in mood often occur gradually following those natural changes, so most people don't make the association. But once you do, a new level of understanding about mood opens up and, with it, potential control.

In this chapter I have reviewed a number of principles of energy variation and the variability of mood. Next we will examine some of the biological bases of mood and, in the last chapter, the best ways of managing our moods as well as counteracting overeating and maximizing exercise.

CHAPTER 8

The Biopsychology of Energy and Tension

O N AN IMPULSE, a friend and I once took a ride on an old mountain ski lift that was temporarily open for summer use. At one point the lift traveled high above the trees, rocks, and vegetation. We were the only ones on the lift and the wind was blowing our chair from side to side—the lift didn't seem all that secure. While looking down I noticed feelings of tension and fear in myself, but the other thing I noticed was that my shoulders were hunched up. I consciously relaxed them and immediately felt less fearful. But after a while I noticed my shoulders were hunched again, and once again the negative emotion was present. The tension I felt with this experience was not a feeling that existed only in my mind; my body—in particular, my muscles—contributed significantly to it. Had I stayed long on that chairlift, I probably would have developed sore shoulders. Back, neck, and shoulder pain are common complaints of people experiencing chronic stress and its accompanying tension. Tight muscles are one way that we react to real or perceived danger.

Like the emotion I experienced on the ski lift, all moods involve the body in some way, and with feelings of tension, the muscles are especially involved. People often think of moods as feelings that exist only in the mind, or they may view these feelings only as reactions of the brain. Instead, diverse systems of the body contribute to what we experience as mood. Moods are a barometer of body states that involve arousal, including fear, anxiety, and a whole host of psychological reactions, some conscious and some not.

Muscle tightness, in particular, is closely associated with feelings of tension, fear, and anxiety, or what I call tense arousal. Thus, in the ski lift episode not only did I feel mildly fearful, but the muscles of my shoulders also were tense, as probably were other muscles of my body. Even mild nervousness entails a certain degree of muscle tension and a particular pattern of muscle activity. If you think about this, as we shall do next in relation to our evolutionary past, you can see why this is so and why it was adaptive to our species.

The Activated Freeze Response

To place this in an evolutionary context, let's consider an experience that might have occurred far back in time, say a hundred thousand years ago. Let's imagine that one of our ancestors is moving through the brush and back to her cave in the evening, when suddenly she hears a threatening growl that is echoing on the canyon walls. This indicates danger, but the location of the possible predator can't be determined. What would she do and how would her body react?

Immediately she would become fully alert and try to determine where the danger lies. Scanning her surroundings with a kind of hypervigilance, she would have difficulty concentrating on anything but the potential danger. Internally, general bodily arousal quickly would occur, preparing her for whatever she might have to do to protect herself. In characterizing her condition, you might think about the well-known *fight-or-flight response*. But in this case fight or flight is not yet appropriate. First, the predator must be located. Before either fight or flight occurs, avoiding detection would be the primary biological imperative.

So what would she do? If she ran wildly through the brush without knowing the whereabouts of the predator, she would immediately increase her chances of being detected and eaten. Her contributions to the gene pool might well be eliminated, so blind fleeing would not be an adaptive response. Instead, she probably would remain frozen where she was, thus reducing the possibility of discovery. But this freeze response would have a characteristic form. Her shoulders would hunch up (remember me on the ski lift), she would crouch forward slightly in a stance protective of vital body parts, her neck and face would tighten, and various other muscles would tighten as well. This is not something that she would have learned to do. The behavior would be programmed long before as part of the evolutionary process. In fact, it is still our first response to danger, and this muscular preparation is optimally effective for whatever emergency might occur, especially when there is uncertainty about what action to take.

Is there a familiar ring to this pattern of muscle tension and inhibition of action, coupled with vigilance and preparatory body arousal? There should be. It is similar to what you might experience in any stressful situation and to what happened to me on the ski lift.

The reaction of our ancestor—and your reaction in a comparable situation—probably would involve a kind of activated freeze response that is programmed for optimal survival. Animals show a similar response. Ethologists are well aware of how a rabbit crouches and freezes, for example, when detecting an approaching fox. They even have a term—flight distance—that denotes the zone beyond which the rabbit will no longer remain frozen. Once the fox approaches closer than that distance, the rabbit will flee—the familiar fight-or-flight response.[1]

When we feel tight muscles because of stress, we are experiencing vestiges of the primitive freeze response. Our life may not be threatened, but a stressful situation will bring out the adaptive patterns of our heritage. Yet the muscle tightness that we experience when we are tense is uncomfortable. We couldn't completely sustain it for very long. That is why we wiggle our foot or tap our fingers or pace, thus unconsciously relieving the tension slightly—a kind of self-regulation. In fact, the foot wiggling and finger tapping are such unerring indications of tension that if you find yourself doing these things you can be sure you are not perfectly calm, even if you think you are. If you want to start trying to remove stress from your day, be on the lookout for these fidgeting movements—they are good indications that you are experiencing tension.

Let's consider this idea a bit further in practical terms. Suppose there is no real danger. You are at your office at work, but you are experiencing a bad mood. You just noticed your shoulders are sore, and you know there must be muscle tension. Remember the principle of body integration I mentioned earlier. The body operates in integrated and holistic patterns, so changing one part of the tension pattern should relieve tension in other ways. Tight muscles are a good place to start, because you have a certain degree of voluntary control over them. Thus relieving your muscle tension, even if only slightly, often can improve your mood. If you can relax your muscles, your tension or anxiety often will be reduced as well. What's more, relieving your muscle tension can occur in the most simple ways, particularly if you are experiencing only mild tension. For example, muscle tension often can easily be relieved with a little stretching or a short walk in which you consciously relax the muscles not necessary for walking and you swing your arms gently to relieve the tension in your shoulders and neck.

I remember a unique example of a simple relaxation technique that I witnessed during a trip to Washington, D.C. I hailed a taxi in rush-hour traffic and was picked up by a cab driven by a wise-looking Middle Eastern man. As we talked, I noticed his unusual calmness, even while he maneuvered quickly through stop-and-go traffic, answered calls on his radio, and carried on a conversation with me at the same time. Then I noticed it—he was driving with one hand while thumbing a circle of beads with the other, one by one. When I asked him about it, he said it relaxed him, and that traffic is never a bother when he uses his beads. As unlikely as it may seem, this kind of small systematic movement can relieve tension in other parts of your body.[2] A similar principle is involved with the soft rubbery objects sold commercially that you squeeze in your hand. They are often billed as stress relievers. Once again we see the example of integration among several body systems. Relaxing one part of the activated freeze response in turn relaxes another part.

You might try something similar the next time you notice you are tense. If you don't have any beads, just slowly twirl a small pencil or toothpick in your fingers for a couple of minutes, or give in to your wiggling foot or tapping fingers by consciously carrying out your impulse, but in a slow and exaggerated form. Do it in such a way as to slowly stretch and relax the muscles that are driving the fidgeting movements.

After a short while, you can observe whether you feel a little better. If you do feel better, and especially if your mood is improved, you will immediately realize how your muscle tension contributes an inordinate amount to how you feel, and it is often unpleasant. You may get a sense that you have been holding yourself back—the freeze pattern—and that the movement was a kind of release. You may also realize how a small change in some muscles can have a spreading effect, reducing tension in other parts of your body.

As another way of relieving mild tension, try taking a short walk, but concentrate on muscle relaxation while you are walking.[3] The walk is an extension of what you already are motivated to do when you feel like pacing. But, as you walk, often you will experience a kind of release—in this case, a release of muscle tension. Short walks, as we have seen, can reduce tension, and this is one of the ways it occurs—releasing inhibition and reducing muscular tension by movement.

The muscle tension that we experience when we are tense, anxious, or nervous is very adaptive as we are preparing to face potential danger. You may recall I said that this is an *activated* freeze. Besides the muscular inhibition, the body is also preparing for action. If we could look inside the body of our prehistoric ancestor, we would see a wide variety of preparatory bodily changes as she gets ready to react to the potential danger. With this kind of arousal, the heart pumps blood more rapidly to areas of the body primed for action, respiration quickens, giving needed oxygen for increased metabolic activity, and more blood glucose pours into the bloodstream to provide fuel for the emergency. Hormones such as adrenaline and cortisol that facilitate arousal are released, hands and feet sweat for efficient action, pupils dilate for the best vision; indeed, throughout the sympathetic nervous system with its far-flung influences there is immediate activation. These kinds of changes occur in the whole body, including an early response by the arousal systems of the brain; for example, such neurotransmitters as norepinephrine and dopamine increase in concentration, thereby activating the nervous system.

These changes come rapidly, some more rapidly than others, but tense arousal occurs in all these ways, and many more. At the same time the body is reacting, we *feel* tense, anxious, or nervous—a complex experience that creates our mood. Our mood is just part of a response that affects both mind and body.

Differences Between Energy and Tension

Arousal is a key concept in understanding our moods. We have just been talking about the type of arousal present in the activated freeze response. But another kind of arousal occurs with exercise. If you are sitting and relaxing, and then you stand and begin to walk briskly, the arousal systems of your body are immediately activated. Some of the same systems that prepare you for action are present whether you are reacting to potential danger or exercising in a pleasant gym. Your cardiovascular and respiratory systems, as well as your general metabolism, for example, underlie physical activity, whether in calm exercise or in preparation for fight or flight. There certainly are some differences in the brain and elsewhere in the body, depending on whether we are experiencing an emergency or pleasant exercise, and we will review some of those shortly, but many elements of arousal are the same because they support vigorous physical activity by the body.

One particular difference between energetic and tense arousal occurs with skeletal muscular activation. While tense arousal involves a kind of "muscular inhibition," energetic arousal entails more directed muscle activity. Thus, when you are very tense your skeletal muscles in effect hold you back—the freeze response—but when you are energized and calm (calm energy) there is none of this inhibition. As an example of calm energy, consider a superb athlete gliding with confidence through a well-practiced routine, showing no hesitation or tension. It looks effortless to us as bystanders, although it undoubtedly required a good deal of trial and error initially. Such world-class routines show us what energetic arousal looks like when there is a minimum of tense inhibition. Such athletes, and some of us weekend sports enthusiasts, can experience calm energy in this form.

If you think about this, you will realize how it makes sense. Energetic arousal is a "go system," as biologists sometimes speak. Tense arousal, on the other hand, is a "stop system."[4] When you feel high energy, it may be hard to sit quietly because physical activity is attractive, and engagement with the outside world is a natural reaction. But when you feel tense, caution and restraint are the natural reactions. These are basically stop and go systems in the most general view, and they balance each other, sometimes bringing us to move, to act, to assert ourselves, and sometimes to be cautious and restrained. Both systems are very adaptive. They aid us to live in a world that requires action but which is sometimes dangerous and requires caution.

These systems involve the whole body. You can notice one good example of tense arousal in your breathing when you are fearful and anxious compared to when you are exercising in a relaxed way and feeling energized. While experiencing fear, you breathe rapidly with short breaths, but with calm exercise you breath more deeply.[5] The short, rapid breaths characteristic of fear probably occur because the muscles surrounding the thoracic cavity are tight in a freeze response, as are many other muscles in your body. Among other effects, this inhibits full lung expansion. But the body needs oxygen when it is aroused, so there is a rapid panting, which enables the lungs to receive the required oxygen. Throughout the body, similar differences can be found in patterns of muscle inhibition compared to directed muscle activity. One of the reasons, by the way, that slowing and deepening your breathing can calm you is that it reduces general arousal in a similar way to the relaxation of muscle tension. Respiration is just one part of a larger pattern that controls the body's arousal.

As you become more aware of how muscle tension interacts with so many of your body's systems, you can begin to use this information to help regulate your moods. For example, you can see why yoga is so effective, with its postures that evolved over hundreds of years as ways of systematically stretching and relaxing muscles. And you can understand why massage can be so effective.

The benefits of massage often are not discussed, perhaps because this form of body and muscle manipulation has been associated with illicit sexual activities, but now there is a considerable amount of research (involving controlled studies with placebo comparisons) demonstrating how massage is effective for everything from migraine headaches, pain relief, and attention deficit disorder/ hyperactivity disorder to enhancing alertness. In addition to these diverse benefits, a number of studies have shown the effectiveness of massage in easing stress, mild depression, and anxiety.[6] Tense arousal, and especially muscle tension, probably underlies many of the negative conditions that massage alleviates.[7]

Massage, yoga, and moderate exercise all indicate how muscle tension plays a central role in mood, and how alleviating muscle tension can help improve our moods. Other aspects of body and brain functioning are also important, as we shall see in the following pages.

Both Body and Brain Direct Our Moods

Many parts of the body and brain are mobilized when we become aroused and feel energetic or when we feel tense. From changes in metabolism, through cardiovascular and respiratory activation, and throughout the brain and nervous system, changes are evident. It is not just one system of the body at work. Instead, it is an integrated pattern with the emphasis on integration. Arousal occurs throughout the body, and mood is part of this because the mind and body are not separated. Because energetic and tense arousal—the underpinnings of mood—are very general reactions, we can't put our finger on any one physiological system and say that this is what causes that kind of arousal. Within the arousal systems of the body, however, certain key elements have been specifically studied in relation to mood. Let me briefly mention several of these important systems that contribute to arousal and mood.

Blood Glucose

Have you ever felt really hungry, so hungry that you were weak? You probably were irritable as well. Children can be great case studies in this respect, as any parent knows. It's no wonder that the exasperated parent gives her crying child something sweet when it isn't time yet for the next meal. She knows that it will work right away to calm the child. The snack probably works in part because it raises blood sugar levels. This fuel that underlies our arousal is pivotal to understanding our moods, as well as our eating habits. Research has demonstrated correlations between increased blood glucose levels, feelings of energy, and reduced tension.[8]

One of the most impressive experimental demonstrations of the relationship between blood glucose and mood was carried out by Ian Deary, Ann Gold, David Hepburn, and their colleagues at the University of Edinburgh in a study of hypoglycemia, an abnormal condition in which the body is unable to maintain enough glucose in the blood to sustain the brain and other vital organ functions. These researchers were experimenting with normal subjects to determine how changing blood glucose would affect mood.[9] Under blind conditions, this group manipulated blood glucose over several hours by using infusions of insulin, which caused blood sugar to drop. The subjects began with a normal state and were driven into a hypoglycemic state, then returned again to a normal state. Insulin and placebo infusions were randomly employed with different people, so subjects could not react according to what they expected.

The effects were dramatic. The investigators were able to drive tension up and energy down by creating a hypoglycemic state. This tense-tired mood state was maintained for an hour. Then, following the reintroduction of normal glucose levels, energy and tension went back to normal. This experiment represents a rare well-controlled demonstration of cause and effect involving physiology and mood. Changing the underlying physiology—in this case, blood glucose levels—caused moods to change from normal to a tense-tired state and back again to normal.[10]

Besides demonstrating an important physiological basis for energy and tension feelings, these findings suggest a reason for the tendency of people to seek sugar snacks when their energy is low and their tension is high (tense tiredness). We already have behavioral evidence for this—we know what people do—but the physiological basis had been difficult to prove before this experiment. The fuel, which is blood glucose, underlies many aspects of bodily arousal, but the anatomical mechanisms of arousal include a far-reaching system that influences our body from head to toe when we become aroused. Let's consider this basic system next.

Autonomic Nervous System

The last time you were frightened, you may have noticed that your hands were sweating, your mouth was dry, and your heart was pounding rapidly. Under great stress, or feeling anxious, you may have noticed that you choked up a bit when you tried to talk, that you got goose bumps, or that the hairs on the back of your neck seemed to stand on end. If you observed these physical reactions for a time, you probably noticed that, as you calmed down, they disappeared. With relaxation, you may even have noticed subtle signs that normal digestion was again under way, after having stopped.

These various arousal and calming reactions of your body are related to activation of the autonomic nervous system and its two branches, the sympathetic and parasympathetic systems. One of the two reciprocal branches of this peripheral nervous system (sympathetic) is responsible for organizing, mobilizing, and expending energy, while the other (parasympathetic) is associated with conserving energy. When we are active and move about, or when we are fearful—indeed, when we feel either energetic or tense—the sympathetic nervous system tends to be activated.

Many different parts of the body are influenced by activation of the sympathetic nervous system, including respiration, heart rate, vasomotor tone, blood pressure, carbohydrate and fatty acid metabolism, and sweat gland activity. As can be seen from these examples among the many components of sympathetic activation, this part of the nervous system is an important element in any response that puts demands on the body—whether stress, exercise, or strong negative and positive emotions.

Parasympathetic activation, on the other hand, generally balances the activity of the sympathetic nervous system. Both systems are usually active at the same time, but their relationship sets the tone of bodily arousal. Parasympathetic effects are quite varied, including such processes as decreased heart rate and increased digestive activity. These and other bodily functions that occur with parasympathetic dominance are present during periods of low tense and energetic arousal, periods associated with energy conservation and recuperation.

In *The Chemistry of Conscious States*, Harvard Medical School professor J. Allan Hobson argues that the autonomic nervous system is the key to energy, mood, and health. He points out that the sympathetic branch of the autonomic system requires us to expend energy that is *ergotropic,* or energy-generating. These effects occur through amine molecules such as norepinephrine. On the other hand, the parasympathetic branch of the autonomic system is *trophotropic,* or energy-conserving. It exercises its calming effects by another neurotransmitter, acetylcholine. Thus, he argues, "the division of labor between the aminergic and cholinergic systems in our brains is mirrored by the division of labor between amines and aceylcholine in the body."[11]

Focusing on sleep, among other things, and especially REM sleep, Hobson makes a good case for why depression—which he calls a disorder of energy—is affected by dysfunctions in sleep. He points out, for example, that depressed people sleep poorly and often complain of feeling tired. Moreover, they are too tired to exercise. Hobson ties these ideas to general health and to immune system functioning. Let's consider a bit further some of these neurochemical influences on arousal.

Hormones and Mood

While the autonomic nervous system produces short and fast-acting physiological responses throughout the body, the effects of hormones, which circulate more slowly in the bloodstream, last longer. We saw the effects of insulin in the example on hypoglycemia and changed blood glucose levels. But a number of other hormones also are associated with our moods—for example, the so-called stress hormones. Deficiencies of some hormones have been specifically associated with mood problems. It is beyond the scope of this book to deal with the effects of the many hormones that have been identified, but I will mention some of the better-known hormonal effects.

Adrenaline and cortisol are sometimes called stress hormones, and both influence arousal responses of the body, but they may have somewhat different effects. Richard Dienstbier of the University of Nebraska identifies two systems of arousal that he believes are similar to energetic and tense arousal.[12] He see these two arousal systems as having different functions and different effects on behavior. In his intriguing theory, Dienstbier describes one arousal system that involves the hypothalamus, a small structure in the central part of the brain, and the sympathetic nervous system, which affects the adrenal medulla, a gland that lies just above the kidneys and is responsible for the release of adrenaline. This adrenaline response results in what Dienstbier calls desirable forms of energy at minimal psychological cost.[13]

In many respects this arousal system appears to parallel energetic arousal. For example, adrenaline levels are closely associated with intensity and effort of exercise, and in a wide variety of ways adrenaline is known to enhance exercise.[14] Moreover, as Dientsbier maintains, this adrenaline response to demand tends to become more efficient with activities such as regular exercise that "toughen" the exerciser.[15] These are exactly the characteristics of energetic arousal.

The second arousal system that Dienstbier identifies appears to be basic to the experience of tension, in that it is activated in stress and emergency circumstances.[16] This system is associated with hypothalamic stimulation of the pituitary, a kind of master gland about the size of a pea that lies at the base of the brain. Among other hormones, the pituitary influences the release of adrenocorticotropin (ACTH), which in turn affects the adrenal cortex, a part of the adrenal gland. In this way, cortisol is released.

Cortisol could play an important role in appetite and in overeating. For example, in her recent book, Pamela Peeke, a physician and National

Institutes of Health researcher, argues that chronic stress results in increased cortisol secretions, which in turn cause utilization of blood glucose stores in the body. In turn, people eat to compensate.[17] It's no accident that cortisol is referred to as a "glucocorticoid" because of its influence on glucose levels, so this makes logical sense as well as being supported by various experimental studies.[18]

A large cortisol response has special implications for understanding mood, because abnormal cortisol levels have been found in people with certain kinds of depression, a condition underlaid by tense tiredness. Excessive cortisol secretions occur in 40 to 60 percent of depressed patients.[19] Many researchers believe that dysregulation of the hypothalamic-pituitary-adrenal system is a biological indicator of mood disorder.[20]

Other hormones also have been linked to depressive disorders. For example, hormone replacement therapy, especially estrogen, has been shown to reduce depression among menopausal women in a number of studies.[21] Low thyroid levels also are associated with depression, and successful treatment results in a beneficial hormone response.[22] Our understanding of the relationship between moods such as depression and hormones is by no means complete, but it is clear that hormones are important. Anyone suffering from depression should have a thorough checkup to rule out physical abnormalities as the cause of their negative moods.

The way that poor eating habits, hormones, and mood interact in relation to changing arousal levels is described by Ronald Hoffman, the physician who is heard widely in his syndicated radio program on health. In *Intelligent Medicine*, he points out how excessive sugar ingestion causes blood glucose to soar, and, as a result, insulin levels rise to sharply reduce this excess.[23] Then, as blood glucose is oversuppressed, adrenal hormones pour out again to raise blood glucose, since this substance is vital for brain and other body sustenance. This roller-coaster ride of sugar highs and lows, as he calls it, leads to powerful mood swings. From this description, we can see how hormones affect moods, but from my previous discussions it is evident that this is an interactive process. Our moods are affected by excessive sugar ingestion, but, in turn, they signal us to eat even more sugar to right ourselves in the quickest way possible. We experience these moods as changing energy and tension levels.

Chemical Imbalance:
Neurotransmitters, Modulators, and Neuropeptides

You undoubtedly have heard depression and other serious mental conditions described as chemical imbalances—as in, "You can't blame him; he has a chemical imbalance." But such comments should not lead you to conclude that only depression, panic disorder, attention deficit, or other serious problems stem from biochemical underpinnings. Actually, all our behaviors, thoughts, and feelings have biochemical substrates—that is, they originate in the biochemistry of the body—and moods are no exception.

At one time physiologists believed that interconnected neurons directly conduct the impulses that run throughout the various parts of the brain and body, and these neurons underlie intelligent human functioning—something like the electrical wiring in a house. Not long ago, however, several important discoveries revealed the existence and function of a large class of neurochemical substances that modulate and make possible communication between neurons, acting at the junctures between neurons—the so-called synaptic clefts—as they are secreted and reabsorbed into cell bodies. These are variously called neurotransmitters (such as norepinephrine, dopamine, acetylcholine, and serotonin), steroids (for example testosterone and estrogen), and peptides (such as endorphins and enkephalins). These substances orchestrate a whole cascade of biochemical events that, in their totality, shape what we feel as moods. In fact, many medical conditions (such as depression) and drugs (like Prozac) influence communication throughout the body by way of effective decreases or increases in these substances.

As our understanding of how the brain and body communicate becomes more complete—really just developed in the last few decades—it has become increasingly clear that the brain operates through the action of these neurochemicals and that their ability to function is facilitated by a large number of receptor sites for these substances throughout the body. As the well-known neuroscientist Candice Pert cogently puts it, "If the cell is the engine that drives all life, then the receptors are the buttons on the control panel of that engine, and a specific peptide . . . is the finger that pushes that button and gets things started."[24]

In her persuasive book *Molecules of Emotion*, Pert makes a strong case for expanding an earlier picture of emotion (and mood) that focused only on various brain structures as causal agents.[25] Instead, she argues that the receptors for informational substances throughout the body make emotions something like "bodymind" phenomena. In other words, emotions do not come only from the brain but also from the rest of the body, where extensive receptor systems result in activation. Marshaling good scientific evidence, she argues that the model that identifies the brain as the exclusive originator of emotion must be replaced by a model in which diverse systems of the body *interact* with the brain to create emotions. This point of view is consistent with what I indicated when describing the way that moods are whole-body phenomena and how they emerge from general bodily arousal. And it is consistent with managing moods by skeletal muscular relaxation, exercise, or other ways of affecting the body. Let's next consider some of the better-known neurochemicals that underlie arousal.

Serotonin, Endorphins, and Other Well-Known Neurochemicals

Serotonin has become the hottest new neurochemical, at least in the public mind. Billed in the popular media as responsible for everything from social status to happiness and flat stomachs, we hear increasingly about this neurotransmitter. The first big public notice came from wonder stories about Prozac, the so-called selective serotonin reuptake inhibitor, or *SSRI* (Zoloft, Paxil, and other drugs came later), which can directly affect serotonin and demonstrate its role in how we feel. The media marveled at the news; here at last was an answer for depression, a new kind of antidepressant that would eliminate the problems with older drugs and cure this serious condition once and for all. Later came reports of benefits for a wide set of problems, including, but not limited to, obsessive compulsive disorder, violent impulse control, premenstrual syndrome, Seasonal Affective Disorder, and even help for troubled children.[26]

What really impressed millions about serotonin, however, was its apparent influence on weight loss. The fen-phen diet, with fenfluramine's effects of increasing serotonin, was bought by millions, and this stampede was quelled only by findings of heart damage from the drug, which eventually caused it to be pulled from the market.

The facts about serotonin are somewhat less glamorous, but nonetheless impressive.[27] In ways that relate to Candice Pert's points, many different kinds of receptors for serotonin have been identified.[28] In biological terms, this neurochemical obviously is extremely important, but just what does it influence, and exactly how does it affect mood and other kinds of behavior? There are lots of hypotheses but no certainty.

In relation to mood, Prozac and other similar drugs that affect serotonin are used by millions of people around the world for depression and a variety of other disorders. The drug appears to have important antidepressant effects, but these should not be overestimated. In one typical study, a little over 60 percent of depressed people were helped by Prozac, but a little under 40 percent got better from a placebo.[29] These kinds of results have led some scientists to note that the best of the antidepressants have only about a 25 percent efficacy, and, what's more, it is argued that these drugs do not work appreciably better in the long term than traditional psychotherapy does.[30]

The positive effects of Prozac and similar drugs on mood as well as the findings of relationships between serotonin and a variety of behavioral effects suggest that this neurotransmitter must play an important part in energetic arousal. For example, we know that energetic arousal underlies wakefulness. Similarly, during wakefulness serotonergic (serotonin) neurons in the brain are most active with general motor activity and other kinds of behavioral arousal.[31] In both animals and humans, exercise elevates brain serotonin.[32] And, once again, energy levels are elevated by exercise, especially moderate exercise.

There are a number of other interesting relationships that involve serotonin and that also suggest energetic arousal. For example, serotonin appears to curtail violent and impulsive behavior, and it seems to stop negative emotional states.[33] In a previous chapter we saw how high energy also appears to suppress tension, and tension is usually a part of these negative emotional states. In another significant respect, we see the way that serotonin seems to suppress eating. This is apparent from the fen-phen diet, and from other studies as well.[34] In a comparable way, increasing energy and the related tension reduction seem to reduce eating as well. Low energy and tension often are the cause of food urges and bingeing, a point I have returned to again and again.

So, is serotonin the neurochemical underpinning of energetic arousal? It's too early to know. This neurochemical system is extremely complex, and we have only begun to understand it. But the evidence seems to point in that direction.

Norepinephrine and dopamine are other important neurotransmitters in the history of research on mood. Norepinephrine, for example, is closely associated with various activated conditions, including the effects of exercise. Similarly, this *catecholamine* is present during wakefulness and stress, and is associated with the effects of stimulant drugs.[35] The early catecholamine theory of depression focused on deficiencies of norepinephrine at important receptor sites in the brain, and although this theory has not been wholly satisfactory as a way of accounting for depression, it remains possible.[36] Also, some antidepressants are thought to be effective because they elevate norepinephrine levels in the brain.

Dopamine, a close cousin of norepinephrine, is also associated with activated states. For a number of reasons this neurotransmitter is likely to be especially important to arousal-related moods. As only one indication of the significance of dopamine to mood, neurons activated by this *amine* appear to be among the most important parts of the brain stem's reticular formation, a brain structure important in bodily arousal. Through its influence in different parts of the brain, dopamine appears to be crucial to various kinds of motor behavior and to circadian rhythmicity.[37]

In other mood-related respects, dopaminergic (dopamine) systems are likely to be important bases of pleasurable aspects of cocaine ingestion and of the kind of pleasurable self-stimulation in the brain that has been demonstrated with implanted electrodes in animals.[38] In general, dopamine could be the base of many positive emotional and mood states. But this neurotransmitter may also be central to brain responses associated with anxiety and stress. Because of these various characteristics, dopamine seems to be related to both energetic and tense arousal.[39]

Endorphins, another interesting group of neurochemical substances, have been much in the news. Popular conceptions hold that they are very important to mood, especially after exercise. Similar in action to opiates—including heroin, morphine, and codeine—the endorphins are thought to reduce stress and bring pleasure in extreme situations.[40] The name *endorphin* is actually short for endogenous morphine. But the existing scientific evidence about endorphins is not consistent with our popular conception. Evidence implying a strong relationship between endorphins and our everyday moods is scant, and there are more likely physiological bases for energy-based positive moods, such as those mentioned earlier, than endorphins. (In a humorous example of how widespread the belief about the positive effects of endorphins has been,

Annette Bening, in the movie *Postcards from the Edge,* tells the Meryl Streep character about her sexual escapades, explaining that she is "in it for the *endolphin* rush.")

The pleasurable feelings we get from intense exercise may be associated with endorphins, but even here the evidence is mixed.[41] And there is little evidence that pleasure from moderate exercise is due to endorphins. So what can we say about endorphins and exercise? On the basis of current scientific research, other explanations for the pleasurable effects of exercise are as likely causes as these brain substances, but the role of endorphins cannot be ruled out from current research findings.

From these various examples of body-brain relationships, we can see what complexity exists underneath our moods, but there is more to say before we are finished with this brief survey of the workings of the body in relation to arousal states. The 1990s was known as the Decade of the Brain, and scientists have been very active in research on this marvelous organ that directs us in so many ways. We look next at the structures of the brain that may be responsible for mood.

Brain Structures Responsible for Arousal and Mood

Reticular Activating System

Researchers are still trying to pinpoint the brain systems that underlie mood, but we do know what regions of the brain are likely to have an important role in the feelings that we experience as moods. Mechanisms of arousal are especially important, and the best-known arousal system is called the reticular formation, or the reticular activating system. The reticular formation is a netlike system of neurons that lies at the base of the brain, and its influence on arousal extends to most higher areas of the brain, as well as into the rest of the body. When we exercise, our whole body is aroused, and the reticular activating system plays an integral part in this pattern. This brain system sends signals up and down the body to amplify stimulation as it occurs in various ways.[42]

Originally, this system was thought only to regulate wakefulness, alertness, and attention, but later research indicated that it has an important influence on the muscular system and motor activity in general. For example, we know that it is involved in the control of breathing and cardiac function and in the coordination of various autonomic activities. Embedded in the reticular formation are cell clusters that produce serotonin, norepinephrine, and dopamine—neurotransmitters that underlie arousal. All these functions are related in essential ways to energetic arousal, an important basis of mood. The reticular activating system is likely to be involved in tense arousal as well, but it is especially significant in the functions associated with energetic arousal.

Limbic System

Another important part of the brain that probably underlies mood is the limbic system.[43] This system of interconnected structures—which include the hypothalamus, hippocampus, and amygdala—lies at the center of the brain, below the cerebral cortex. It influences many vital functions of the body (for example, the autonomic and somatic areas) and also the cerebral cortex, the portion of the brain that is most evolved in humans. Neuropsychologists sometimes joke that the limbic system regulates the four F's of motivated behavior: fleeing, feeding, fighting, and . . . *sexual behavior.* A great deal of research underscores the importance of this brain system in emotional behavior, especially in regard to the fear responses that are so much a part of tense arousal, and thus of mood. Fear and anxiety are mediated by various parts of the brain, including the prefrontal cortex and the endocrine connections of the hypothalamus, but the limbic system plays an integral part.

A sophisticated view of the limbic system was provided in Joseph LeDoux's excellent book, *The Emotional Brain.*[44] In it he details the special role of the amygdala as one of the most important parts of the limbic system in mediating emotional behavior, particularly fear and related emotions. Since fear is an integral part of what I call tense arousal, his views clearly are relevant. He argues that the central arousal systems produce rather nonspecific activation of the brain, but fear-related stimuli depend for their effect on interactions between the amygdala and the acetylcholine-containing systems nearby in the forebrain. Immediate fear reactions depend on activation of the amygdala, and usually they also involve working memory (important for interpretation of the danger). But sustained feelings of fear require activation of the arousal systems, as well as feedback from other parts of the body, in his view. Sustained fear is similar to a mood.

Given the likelihood that many parts of the brain contribute to both energy and tension, it is too simple to assert that the reticular activating system mediates energetic arousal and the limbic system mediates tense arousal. Because the types of behavior that these systems influence are so central to the two kinds of arousal, however, I would say that the reticular activating system must be involved in a major way with energetic arousal, as is the limbic system with tense arousal.[45]

Cerebral Cortex

The cerebral cortex is a thin layer of cells that is folded and deeply grooved. If you spread it out flat, it would be about two and a half square feet. It wraps around the more primitive structures of the brain. We have known for some time that this part of our brain, which is newest in evolutionary terms, controls thinking and other advanced human functioning. But now it is increasingly apparent that it may play a role in our moods as well—not in the way you would assume, by influencing our thoughts about things, but more directly.

This mood function became evident some years ago when doctors observing stroke patients noticed that some types of stroke left their patients feeling depressed.[46] Depression of this kind occurred to a much greater degree when the damage to the brain centered in the front of the cortex on the left side than when the stroke damaged other brain areas. It seemed as though that particular area of the cortex must have something to do with mood, and especially depression.

One of the newest chapters in the search for the seat of emotional activity in the brain involves research in which scientists use electronic sensors to determine where electrical activity occurs in the cerebral cortex, and whether a particular pattern of activity is related to people's moods. These studies seem to indicate that reduced activation of the left side of the cortex (left hemisphere) sets up a kind of asymmetry between the two sides of the brain. That is, damage in the left hemisphere results in greater activation in the right hemisphere, because in normal states the two sides would otherwise balance each other.[47] Conversely, left-hemisphere asymmetry is associated with neutral or positive emotions. This intriguing theory seems to indicate that our brains are organized to cause positive and negative moods and that the two kinds of moods balance each other by way of the underlying hemispheres of the brain.

Consider how this might work. Nathan Fox, Richard Davidson, An-

drew Tomarken, and others argue an interesting model of cerebral differ-
entiation in which so-called approach tendencies occur with left asymmetry, and avoidance or withdrawal tendencies with right asymmetry.[48] In
their view, approach tendencies are associated with what biologists sometimes call heightened appetitive (from *appetite)* or incentive motivation.
Animals that are especially responsive to rewards or positive stimuli are
sometimes described as having strong approach or appetitive tendencies.
On the other hand, these scientists argue that right frontal activation can
be tied to protective and defensive tendencies.[49]

If you consider the essence of what is involved in appetitive and defensive patterns of behavior, you can see the strong parallel with energetic
and tense arousal. Feelings of energy motivate approach tendencies, while
tension feelings are associated with avoidance, withdrawal, caution, or
inhibition. In other words, when we feel energetic we want to move forward, we want to act, we want to approach. As I described it earlier,
energy is a "go" feeling. But when we feel tense we aren't motivated to
approach. Instead, the message that our moods are relaying is to stop and
evaluate the situation before acting. Caution and inhibition represent a
kind of "stop" tendency.

In the case of our prehistoric ancestor experiencing the freeze
response that I described earlier, when she heard a sound that indicated
danger, the tension she felt would have stopped her. She would have
become cautious and careful. Approach, which in this case would mean
moving toward her abode and otherwise doing the things she was doing,
would not be her primary motivation. Instead, her primary motivation
would be to stop in a frozen stance and to avoid detection by a possible
predator. Taking the most broad perspective, it is apparent from this the
way that stop and go tendencies balance each other in a general kind of
way. Stop moods like tension seem to balance go moods like energy, and
the two may come from the two sides of the cerebral cortex.

From all of this, you can see why it appears that the cerebral cortex has
a vital role in understanding mood. This association is not surprising,
since we have already seen how thoughts and moods are closely con-
nected, but the relationship appears to be even more basic than that.
Before you think about this in too simplistic a way, however, bear in mind
an additional point related to cerebral asymmetry. There are complex
interactions between the lower brain structures and cerebral cortical

processes, and therefore, mediation of energetic and tense arousal at the level of the reticular and limbic systems undoubtedly interacts with cerebral mediation. All this, in turn, is made possible by biochemical messenger systems that operate throughout the body.

As we survey the body and brain in our search for the underpinnings of mood and arousal, the picture is one of continuous interrelationships. Energetic and tense arousal—positive and negative moods—are very general systems. Their origins lie throughout our underlying physiology, and they have clear-cut biological utility. Coming back to a message I have stressed in this book, our moods are signal systems of general bodily functioning. They tell us of health and illness, of danger and safety, of optimal and poor times for functioning. And they influence us to eat and not to eat, as well as to exercise and not to exercise.

Because our moods and the various bodily systems that they represent are so integrated, a great deal of control and management are possible through understanding these interrelationships. In the next chapter, I will summarize some of the most important points made in this book about overeating and exercise, and then turn to how we might best apply this knowledge to manage and control ourselves.

CHAPTER 9

Managing Your Mood

T O SUM UP WHAT WE HAVE LEARNED up to this point about mood
and how it relates to obesity and lack of exercise:

- Our moods determine our enjoyment of life. We habitually attempt
  to self-regulate these moods, sometimes consciously, but often we
  aren't aware of how much we do this. Scientific studies show the most
  common self-regulation methods—ways that people try to avoid
  feelings of depression and anxiety or try to get into a good mood.
  This process works like self-medication, and it involves activities as
  well as substances. We know that some of the things people do to
  improve their mood are effective, but many only cause greater mood
  problems.
- Two of the most basic ways that people self-regulate their moods are
  eating and physical activity. Understanding these methods of self-
  regulation helps to answer the important public health question of
  why obesity has been increasing at alarming rates, particularly in the
  last two decades. Closely related is the question of why people are
  not exercising enough.
- The mood life of Americans has gradually become more negative in
  the last twenty years, with eating and exercise patterns probably
  affected. Stress is experienced in ever-increasing amounts and, like
  obesity, now stands in epidemic proportions. In addition, nationwide
  statistics show mounting episodes of serious depression and even

greater amounts of moderate depression. Anxiety, substance abuse, and other mood problems are also on the rise.

- As we seek answers for problems of growing obesity and lack of exercise, we should focus on reliable findings from many scientific studies that are often overlooked. Understanding mood is the key. We must look at the exact moods that influence overeating or avoidance of exercise each time they occur, rather than focusing on important but less immediate causes such as heredity, type of diet, or version of exercise program. It is the accumulation of many incidents of mood-driven overeating and inactivity that results in obesity or in chronic avoidance of exercise.

- The origins and functions of moods that influence eating and exercise are clarified by the latest scientific analyses. Careful studies have revealed conditions under which overeating occurs—tiredness and tension, two key elements of mood—and these same states reduce the likelihood of exercise, the very activity that can counteract negative moods. These negative mood elements are especially magnified by stress, as well as being influenced by other natural processes.

- Through years of learning and conditioning, we are motivated to overeat in even mild states of low energy and tension, and we form strong eating habits, sometimes dysfunctional ones. This is especially true with consumption of good-tasting foods that are laden with sugars and fats—foods that provide an immediate energy boost. Food urges often occur without awareness of the real causes, which derive from moods. The same conclusions can be drawn about emotional eating, in which causal conditions like depression, anxiety, anger, boredom, and loneliness are implicated, all showing varying degrees of low energy and tension.

- Tension and tiredness usually underlie negative moods, and they cause overindulgence as people attempt to self-regulate these deficits, but sometimes overeating occurs simply as a way of enhancing an already positive mood. Studies of relapse when diets are broken and exercise programs abandoned clearly identify energy and tension as fundamental influences, however. While negative moods most strongly affect the eating patterns of certain types of people—for example, those who diet regularly—most people's eating is affected by their moods to some degree.

- The growing scientific literature on exercise clearly shows how different intensities and forms of exercise affect mood and, in turn, eating. For example, moderate exercise raises energy; more intense exercise reduces tension. Both improve mood. Important for weight control is the little-known fact that moderate exercise, systematically applied, can temporarily reduce appetite. Increased exercise not only improves the balance of energy-in versus energy-out that controls weight, but it aids appetite suppression through its effect on mood.

- We all seek optimal energy in our waking lives. Energy is the vitality of our being. When we self-regulate our moods, we engage in a kind of pleasure seeking that is closely related to energy. Food and physical activity are two important ways through which this occurs, and people can turn to one or the other for pleasure. In the most general respect, obese people self-regulate their pleasure with food more than with physical activity. As people grow older, their energy balance gradually shifts as they get less exercise and eat the same amount of, or more food. Coupled with the body's naturally decreasing metabolism, this can result in increasing weight.

- Understanding the operation and function of moods is vital to controlling eating and exercise. Moods are signal systems of general body arousal, and they indicate everything from physical to psychological health. Food and exercise affect energy and tension naturally and directly, but other influences include sleep, time of day, mental activities, and stress. Thinking, too, affects mood, just as mood affects thinking.

- The biology and biochemistry of moods are not fully understood, but what we do know shows that the moods we experience are interrelated with many systems of the body. Energetic arousal is a kind of "go" system, while tense arousal signals "stop" and caution. Muscle tension and other parts of the body that are responsible for general arousal are especially important to understand when managing moods. Unlike negative moods that cause overeating, the most optimal moods involve high energy and an absence of tension. This feeling of calm energy perfectly facilitates exercise and appetite control and, once understood, is fully achievable by everyone.

The Best Strategy for Eating Healthy
and Maintaining an Exercise Program

If our collective mood is worsening as life becomes increasingly more rapid, complex, and stressful, should we just give in to the negative effects, including growing obesity and inactivity? Or should we take action and make a change? The choice is ours, but it requires effort. Fully confronting the negative moods that drive overeating and lack of exercise isn't easy. It takes a commitment to observe and understand your moods, as well as to manage them systematically. But the benefits of mood management include a natural kind of weight control and regular exercise that is a pleasure rather than a burden. Moreover, the greatest benefits probably occur with happiness and self-fulfillment, as well as an absence of debilitating depression and anxiety—the problems that plague so many. Furthermore, the biggest mood changes occur at first, so with effective management you can expect substantial improvements at the beginning.

Awareness

We saw how a decline in energy and the accompanying rise in tension are associated with food urges, and it is highly likely that the resulting tense tiredness motivates self-regulation, often in the form of overeating. These changes in mood occur naturally, and they are quite predictable. With the ability to predict comes the power to control. Since people differ in exactly when and under what conditions these mood shifts occur, however, effective management requires sharpening awareness of moods, and this is where self-study becomes extremely valuable. It is essential to become familiar with the full range of your variations in energy and tension, not just the highest and lowest levels. In other words, it is important to recognize subtle variations in your moods.

This recognition of basic mood changes requires practice. When people are under stress it is easy to overlook mild tense tiredness—the kind of mood that breaks down resolve and inevitably leads to broken diets and skipped exercise. While extreme tension is recognized by most, mild tension becomes second nature to the person who works long hours under constant deadlines. And yet the effects of this almost undetectable state eventually emerge. Energy depletion and tension manifest themselves as food urges and binges or as an inability to get to the gym. But the underlying mood causes often go unnoticed.

Once you become familiar with how your body reacts to different energy and tension states throughout the day, you will begin to understand more clearly how these states affect your behavior. Making behavioral changes through awareness of underlying psychological dynamics is a time-tested process in psychology. Most systems of psychotherapy emphasize the importance of awareness. Once a person understands the way that psychological events are strung together—and this means, among other things, seeing the way feelings and thoughts arise and influence one another—it becomes more possible to modify and change behavioral outcomes. With this kind of awareness you can activate and fully use your powerful cognitive system to control your body.

In my experience, once intelligent people become aware of the way these moods affect negative habits, they usually can figure out ways to manage their behavior. Partly, this is because moods are strongly influenced by energy and tension levels, and most people have a good deal of experience with these states. It is apparent that the real problem in managing mood-driven behavior is lack of awareness of the underlying nature of moods and poor understanding of how moods affect behavior. Once these dynamics are understood, intelligent people can bring to bear their often considerable storehouse of experience to manage the problem. Awareness is the key.

Over the years I have found that several kinds of self-study especially sharpen awareness of moods and their effects on behavior. These studies include discriminating daily mood changes and focusing on critical times of day, analyzing the sensations of hunger and satiety in relation to mood, as well as studying the way mood, exercise, and relaxation interact. These exercises are all aimed at recognizing how energy and tension states, which are so basic to our familiar moods, come to drive our self-regulatory behavior, sometimes obviously but more often in subtle ways. Moreover, these self-studies enable us to take account of our many individual differences. After completing these studies, people can tailor a method of self-regulation of their moods for their own temperament and experience.

I believe these exercises can lead to an understanding of why we overeat and avoid exercise, and thus can lead to greater self-fulfillment. But don't trust my word alone—let's consider these self-studies.

Becoming Aware of Daily Cycles of Energy and Tension

Recall that, on average, people experience low energy on awakening, with gradually increasing energy to a daily high point at late morning or early afternoon. A dip then occurs in late afternoon, and a subpeak in the early evening, before energy declines to its lowest point of the day just before sleep. Although this is the typical cycle, there are lots of individual differences, so it is important to study yourself. Over the years in our research I have observed cycles in which the highest hours in daily energy occur in the morning ("morning people") or later in the afternoon, and occasionally in the evening ("night people," who tend to have afternoon or late hour peaks). These high- and low-energy times are more or less the same day after day, although they certainly are influenced by unusual events on any one day—say, a late evening out on a weekday.

One of the most important elements in this daily pattern is the low energy that occurs predictably each day. Studies show that at these low-energy times people are particularly driven to snack. These are also periods when binges can occur. What's more, at these low-energy times, the prospects of exercise can be unpleasant. Even the most determined plans for exercise can be sabotaged by fatigue. A self-study of your personal energy cycle can yield great benefits in understanding why your diet gets broken, and the information gained can be used to plan alternatives to overeating. This analysis will also tell you why intended exercise at certain times of day easily can lead to failure, but at other times of day you will succeed.

I mentioned this study in Chapter 7, but let me remind you about it here and describe it more fully. Use a diary, a spiral notebook that you keep with you that allows you to rate your energy and tension at each hour of the day. Or photocopy the chart in the appendix to this book. Your task is to rate your energy and tension when you awaken and continue to make these ratings at the top of every waking hour. It will take only a few seconds for each rating, but you should continue the ratings throughout the day. (All told, the self-ratings should take less than an hour.) You might even want to remind yourself by setting your watch to beep every hour.

Choose a typical day for the study, when you awaken and go to sleep at about the same time as you do on most days, and then repeat the same procedure on two more typical days. If anything out of the ordinary happens that makes you very anxious or excited that day, stop making ratings and begin again on another day. Your averages for energy and tension for all three days should then be plotted on a graph (use different colors for energy and tension). With this procedure, you will get a picture of your natural biopsychological energy cycle.

Looking over your graph, you will be able to determine which hours require special vigilance about overeating. These times won't always hold, but by and large they will be your critical periods day after day. You will also be able to judge when exercise is easiest, or at least understand why exercise is hard at certain times of day. The low-energy times of day are when you can expect rising tension, and these are periods when food urges often occur. Exercise is more difficult during low-energy hours and more appealing at high-energy times—particularly times of high energy and low tension, a combination that especially facilitates physical activity and some kinds of sedentary cognitive tasks.

This basic procedure for becoming aware of how your energy and tension shift throughout the day in a natural pattern is an extremely valuable way of sharpening your awareness of the critical feelings that underlie much of your behavior. Moreover, the information about yourself that you gain with this kind of study will be invaluable for understanding many aspects of your behavior that may have been mysterious in the past. For example, in addition to eating and exercise tendencies, you will be able to judge when negative and depressing thoughts are most likely to emerge—at times when you are tense and fatigued.

If you want to learn even more about yourself regarding eating, you can extend the ratings of energy and tension levels by adding a separate rating of your urge to snack. Soon it will become apparent how these tendencies to eat are related to energy and tension patterns—the relationships will jump out at you. These constituents of mood are like signal systems of our needs for food.

A few more words about tension ratings: I have found that some people remain unaware of their low-level tension because they are always a little tense, so they feel as though they are perfectly calm when in fact they are not. A session or two of biofeedback, focusing on muscle tension in parts of the body such as your neck, jaw, or back, would demonstrate this immediately. In the absence of biofeedback, you should think about this if your tension ratings are usually at the lowest level but you nervously wiggle your foot or continually move your legs while you are seated. These are sure signs of low-level tension. Biting your nails, twirling your hair, playing with a pencil, or other nervous mannerisms are also sure signs of at least some tension. In one study we did of how college students recognize their tension, we found that some people use impatience and irritability to notice when they are tense. Once you begin to focus on these indications of tension, and continue to make your ratings, this internal state will become much more apparent. You will have increased awareness of your tension, which will allow you to understand why many bad habits persist.

Mood Influences on Food Urges, Hunger, and Satiation

A second kind of study that can reveal your eating patterns involves focusing first on your food urges outside of planned meals. This will make you more aware of how various social interactions, sights and smells of food, and a wide variety of other situations can have a great effect on your tendencies to eat unnecessarily. I predict you will find not just that different circumstances seem to control your eating behavior, but that the degree of control is influenced by changing mood patterns. Sometimes the sight or smell of food can influence you a little, but the urge to eat isn't that strong. On other occasions, however, your behavior may seem driven, and it is here that mood can be especially significant.

For this study, carry a diary in which you systematically describe your food urges unrelated to a planned meal, and at the same time rate your energy and tension levels. When you want to eat in ways that you shouldn't (for example, when you have eaten sufficient food recently), describe the urge in as much detail as you have time for, and also make mood ratings. Focusing on your food urges just a few times will make you much more aware of their complexity and how they are related to your moods.

I think you will find that this process results in an increase in awareness about important distinctions in these urges, even if it doesn't seem as though it will when you first consider the exercise. For example, you may note that the most troublesome urges occur at certain hours of the day—

for example, the late afternoon and evening. You may also find that some energy-intensive foods become more attractive at certain times.

This type of study will also alert you to social settings that may be especially influential in driving your food urges, and you may get an idea of how subconscious learning about these things works—for example, learning that negative moods have driven you in the past to eat good-tasting foods in certain situations and circumstances, and your mood improved afterward. Later, when the context is similar, even the vestiges of those negative moods can stimulate food urges. Various characteristics of the situations can become closely associated with the moods that were involved, so these characteristics also stimulate your food urges. Sights of food and people eating, certain smells, and even seemingly unrelated thoughts are examples. You may feel like one of Pavlov's dogs, but this kind of thing happens to everyone, and becoming aware of it is an important key to control.

After studying your food urges for a time, next extend this study to what you feel when you are hungry for planned meals. Also, during your meals, study what you feel like when you have eaten enough. Sometimes this feeling may extend past satiation to feeling stuffed. As before, of course, rate your energy and tension at the same time as you are describing your hunger and satiation. Once again, a diary can be used for these entries, and you can use five- or seven-point scales for energy and tension ratings. You may be surprised by what you learn from this kind of self-study.

Research on how people know when they are hungry indicates that the most common indications of hunger involve gastric sensations (stomach growls and aches), feelings of weakness, and sometimes tension.[1] Sensations vary, of course, depending on the degree of hunger, and with extreme hunger people experience what Jean Mayer and his associates at Harvard called the familiar triad of irritability, nervousness, and tension (notice the mood relations).[2] Mayer also found that people felt cheerfulness and excitement at the beginning of the meal, to be gradually replaced by feelings of calm contentment. Sleepiness was also frequently reported, but I believe that this occurs when too much has been eaten.

Because you are focusing on energy and tension levels at the same time that you focus on hunger, you will begin to make subtle discriminations. You will see what part of your hunger is driven by your moods, and what part is associated with a physiological or metabolic deficit arising from lack of nutrition.

Satiation is a bit more difficult to recognize easily, but it is very important to be familiar with what healthy satiation feels like if you wish to avoid overeating. When you become good at recognizing satiation, you will be able to eat just enough to satisfy your body's physiological needs and not be overly full. This simple discrimination can save a lot of calories in the long run.

Try to banish from your mind those instructions to "clean your plate!" and stop eating when your tension has been relieved and your energy has been raised to pleasant levels, not when tiredness sets in.[3] Making such fine discriminations may require eating more slowly, and periodically monitoring your level of satisfaction. There is a certain period of time between food ingestion and the psychological effects being registered in consciousness. Wolfing down your food undoubtedly short-circuits this process of self-awareness and can result in overeating, whereas eating more slowly and pausing from time to time gives your body time to react and register in consciousness, thus making you aware of when to stop eating. This will be a fine-tuning process that requires observing when hunger strikes again after eating, so that you eat enough to avoid getting hungry too soon after the last meal. This may mean switching to more frequent, smaller meals.

Use your moods—energy and tension levels—to tell you the best strategy. The type and amount of food you eat should help you maintain energy during the peak times of day and avoid tension that occurs because you need food. If you pay attention not only to your feelings of satiation while eating but also to the way tense tiredness diminishes with food, you will soon see what part of your eating and overeating is mood-related and what part is due to more basic nutritional needs.

Personal Problems and Low Self-Esteem

A third kind of study involves focusing on troubling problems, lapses in self-esteem, and the effects of these things on your eating tendencies. This study is especially valuable if you have noticed that whenever you think about your problems, or whenever you start to think badly about yourself, foods urges crop up. Even if you haven't noticed that association, you will probably see a link between troubling thoughts and variations in your self-esteem. Once again, the aim here is to sharpen awareness that may have become dulled over the years.

Again using your diary, whenever you notice negative thoughts, note what they are, rate your energy and tension levels, and make a note of whether you have a food urge. One thing you may learn from this study is that, if you become very tense, food is not at all attractive to you, but with just moderate degrees of tension, food urges occur. This is a common pattern. If you pay attention to these states over an hour or so, you may also learn that when you first become upset (tense) you are not hungry, but a while later you become exceptionally hungry.

Observing your mood associations with personal problems and thoughts of low self-esteem has a great deal of value outside of reactions to food and exercise. Many negative and depressing thoughts can be understood with reference to how much sleep you recently had, whether you have been sedentary for some time, when you ate last, the time of day, your general health, and other similar matters.[4] This kind of assessment is an index of tense tiredness, and all sorts of negative thinking and depressing thoughts are directly related to these deficits.

On a practical level, this information can be extremely valuable if for no other reason than that it helps you to stop thinking about problems at certain times. We know that negative thoughts are associated with bad moods, and cognitive mood therapies are to some extent based on this association. Thus, as a way of managing mood, it makes sense not to think about your problems. This is extremely difficult but not impossible. Start by trying not to think about them when you recognize that your energy is low and your tension is high because of one of the above deficits.

Extending this relationship between negative moods and thoughts about eating, another measure of eating control is suggested. We know from careful research that overeating is often preceded by thoughts about the desired food. And it is likely that this relationship is made more persistent by tense tiredness. Thus, anything that contributes to tense-tiredness can make thoughts about food more powerful motivators. So, if you find that you start thinking about diet-breaking foods and you realize that you haven't had enough sleep the night before, or you have been sitting and especially inactive for a long time, you may come to realize how tense tiredness is driving your thoughts. This awareness can give you an idea of how those thoughts can be controlled—in these cases, by getting enough sleep and physical activity.

Depression, Anxiety, Boredom, Loneliness, and Anger

We have seen that negative moods precede overeating, but also that individual differences can be important, so you should become especially aware of how you react to your negative moods. Feelings of depression, loneliness, or boredom are indications of mood and have a great deal of influence over your urge to eat.

In the same way as ratings were made in the previous exercises, you may wish to focus on your feelings of depression (or other moods) and how they influence your desire to eat. Again, a five- or seven-point scale can be used to rate your mood in a diary that you carry with you. Along with each rating, note your interest in food and exercise. The context in which these negative moods occurs is often meaningful, so you should pay attention to that as well. Do particular events usually occur before the mood, and do certain thoughts usually precede your mood momentarily? As before, factors such as time of day and how active or sedentary you are can be important antecedents to your moods as well.

If you have already done ratings of your energy and tension changes with time of day, after doing this study you may notice how your depressed feelings closely parallel energy and tension at predictable times, and this can be a great insight. Previously, you may have been aware that sometimes you felt depressed and sometimes you did not, but you attributed these occasional feelings to events or even to something uncontrollable in your mind. Seeing a parallel with naturally changing energy patterns can give you an understanding that your feelings of depression are not random, but tend to occur at certain times. We have some control over these energy and tension states. (While you are doing these observations, if you notice that your depressed feelings are continuous and long-lasting, you should consult a physician, psychologist, or psychotherapist. This exercise is meant to focus on feelings of moderate depression, not more serious clinical states.)

Carefully studying their depression and food urges, many people will recognize something like the following. Feelings of depression become apparent, often in the context of low energy at certain times of day or thoughts about personal problems. Thoughts about food soon follow. This may stimulate an internal dialogue in which you recite dietary prohibitions previously made: "I promised myself not to eat that." And in the sequence of thoughts that rapidly occurs, thoughts of hopelessness appear: "Why bother with my diet when I am so worthless anyway?" This will drive you into a worse mood. You will eat the food, and the act of eating is proof positive that you have no control, thus wiping out any vestiges of self-discipline. Binge eating can follow—maybe not a whole cake, but two or three pieces when one would have been plenty. From this scenario you can see the complex influences of mood and thoughts on undesirable habits.

Patterns of moods and thoughts are the common catalysts of dietary failure, and they make perfect biopsychological sense. Feelings of depression are unpleasant, and they motivate escape in the form of self-regulation. And since this is a low-energy state, energy-generating food is the obvious remedy, although the basis of this motivation may be largely unconscious. The food makes you feel good, even if only temporarily, and the good feelings counteract the depression. Just understanding this sequence can give us some control over our eating.

Reactions to Stress

It's worth keeping a stress journal from time to time as a way of becoming aware of how much stress you are experiencing. When elevated stress in your life becomes the norm, it begins to feel perfectly natural. But whether you realize it or not, you are reacting to that stress, and poor eating habits and excessive consumption of energy-intensive foods are only some of the ways that you may be self-regulating.

To at least sample the pressure you are under, keep a diary in which you regularly rate your degree of stress (perhaps a five- or seven-point scale, from the most stress you usually feel to the least). The time you spend focusing on these ratings is critical, and the more often you can do them the more your understanding will improve. If you are experiencing time pressures, however, it may be unrealistic to do hourly ratings. You may have to settle for a time each day when you rate your degree of stress in the previous period. In the evening, before you become too tired, is a good time to rate your day. Your understanding will become more acute if your ratings encompass changes in stress. These variations make you focus on differences, and that is always a good way of making discriminations. Thus, observing yourself for a month or so when different days are more or less stressful will give you a sense of how your stress changes and what effects these changes have.

At the same time as you do these ratings, rate your energy and tension levels as best you can. This will be less satisfactory than making momentary ratings, but at least you can get an idea of how you were feeling earlier. While you are making your stress and mood ratings for the previous period, note what you can about appetites for particular foods and your interest in exercise. Pay attention to fast foods, including not only what you ate but what you had a particular hankering for. The times that you actually exercised in this period are important, but even if you didn't, you should try to rate your interest in and your avoidance of exercise.

You may be surprised by the degree to which your desire for food and exercise changes with stress. Your eating habits are particularly subject to the influence of stress. Studies have shown that fast foods are eaten more frequently when people are under stress, and this includes not only the amount of fast foods but also increased interest in energy-intensive foods—those with high sugar and fat content. Similarly, consistent exercise is less likely when stress is high, not only because you have less time, but because when your resources are drained, exercise becomes less attractive.

How Do You Self-Regulate Your Moods?

As we have seen in earlier chapters, we all self-regulate our moods in various ways to avoid unpleasant feelings and to enhance pleasant ones. This process occurs almost unconsciously. But focusing on this tendency in such a way as to bring it into full consciousness gives you a certain degree of control. Eating is one of the ways that people self-regulate, but other ways are also common. If mood regulation motivates us to eat, alternative ways of self-regulating that mood can be substituted. With awareness comes control.

In this self-study, use a diary in which you note your tendencies to do things to make yourself feel better, especially over time. When you are feeling out of sorts, what do you usually do? Also, if you are feeling okay, but you want to feel even better, what thoughts and actions do you take? Understanding your usual modes of self-regulation can be very enlightening.

In our research, some form of social interaction was the most common way people tried to feel better (to self-regulate mood)—especially women. Another frequent method was to change their thoughts—to try to think positively, concentrate on something else, or give themselves a pep talk. Music was another common method. A variety of other behaviors were commonly used in varying amounts.

About a third of people admitted that they usually eat something when they are in a bad mood, but I suspect that eating is even more widespread for at least occasional mood regulation. Thus, while some people are almost guaranteed to be obese by their usual ways of self-regulating their moods, others may just be overweight for reasons they don't understand. They don't always eat to self-regulate their moods, but often enough they do, and gradually increasing weight is the consequence.

Another third of people indicated that they exercise when they are in a bad mood, and they have chosen the best form of self-regulation. Your usual mode of self-regulation determines your balance of eating and physical activity as a means of managing your energy and tension.

Your Exercise Time

Abundant physical activity is essential for weight management, as well as for physical and psychological health. So, why do so many people resolve to exercise regularly but ultimately fail? One important reason, I believe, is that they are choosing the wrong times to exercise—"throwaway" times, when they don't have the energy to do anything else. This may be necessary because of their busy schedules, but it reduces the likelihood that they will be successful at a long-term exercise commitment.

Low energy makes exercise unattractive, but when your energy is high you are more likely to want to exercise. These are biological givens. So if you wish to make regular exercise a part of your long-term lifestyle, choose times to do it when your energy is high. And if you want to know why you don't exercise, pay attention to your negative moods at the time when exercise is scheduled.

For this self-study, monitor your moods and thoughts in the hour before you intend to exercise and during the time when the exercise is to occur. In addition to the usual ratings of energy and tension, note how you are thinking about the prospective exercise. And, of course, pay attention to matters such as whether you need sleep, what you have eaten (especially if it was a big helping of some junk food that made you tired), what time of day it is, and so on. If you find that you usually have naturally occurring tense tiredness at the time that you are planning to exercise, your avoidance of exercise should be no mystery.

As a second part of this study, try paying attention to your mood when you actually feel like exercising. Even if this hits only occasionally, when does this feeling occur? What are your levels of energy and tension like? Do you feel like exercising at a certain time of day, and is the feeling related to what you have eaten? Is your interest in physical activity related to how much sleep you have had and your level of stress? These are all related to your energy and tension and will give you some understanding of why exercise is sometimes attractive and sometimes not.

Effects of Exercise on Mood

We have seen how physical activity and feelings of energy are integrally related. Moderate exercise raises energy temporarily, and physical conditioning through long-term exercise leads to sustained levels of higher energy. Of course, too much physical activity can reduce energy, but the low levels of physical activity that modern people maintain usually do not reach that point of diminishing energy, except in short-term exertion or in conjunction with health problems. Exercise also can reduce tension, although this mood relationship with exercise is not as clear as the exercise-energy association. In any event, the mood effects of exercise have been evident in study after study. Therefore, in managing your moods it is essential to be fully aware of how physical activity affects you. This information is vital to self-control.

Begin your self-study of exercise effects on mood with moderate exercise, because that is where the exercise-energy association is most evident. In Chapter 3, I described a self-study with walking. Let me review it here and use the same basic procedure to suggest other studies as well. Do this self-study on several occasions when you have been sitting for a while and feeling tired, especially if you have been sitting for an hour or so. Rate your energy on a five- or seven-point scale. Next, get up and go out for a ten-minute brisk walk. Try to walk about the speed you would if you were late for an appointment, but without the anxiety you might feel if that were true. Breathe rhythmically and deeply. Try to remain fairly erect, but relax the muscles of your body that are not necessary for walking or for swinging your arms naturally. When you finish the walk sit down and relax for a minute or two, then rate your energy again. You might also rate your tension before and after the walk, but changes in tension usually are less evident than changes in energy.

You probably will find that you feel more energetic on the second rating compared to the first, but there could be individual differences. For example, an Olympic walker may feel little effect from only ten minutes. But if this kind of moderate exercise affects you, anytime that you want to raise your energy you can simply go for a walk.

We saw in Chapter 5 an example related to appetite in which raising your energy can be very useful in counteracting an urge to eat. Recall that moderate exercise—in one study, a brisk five-minute walk—significantly reduced the appetite for a sugar snack. You can take advantage of this information not only to counteract the peak of an urge to snack but also to understand the underlying nature of these urges, particularly the influence of low energy on your appetite. We know that people on a diet experience peaks and troughs in their urge to eat, and if they can withstand the urge for a little while it often diminishes. If a small amount of moderate exercise will reduce your urge to eat, even for a short time, you may be able to stay on that diet.

To do this experiment on yourself, the next time you experience an urge to eat when you think you have eaten enough recently, rate your urge on a five- or seven-point scale, and also rate your energy and tension. Then take a five-minute brisk walk. If you are in an office building, walk down the hall, up the stairs, down that hall, down those stairs, and so on. This is good exercise because you get to walk, climb, and descend, thus activating a variety of muscles. Since you will be walking briskly, the people you encounter will just think you are walking to an appointment, and you won't have to explain to them that you are doing research (until the second or third time anyway). After five minutes, rate your urge and your energy and tension once again. If you are like the majority of subjects in our research, you will experience a reduction in urge accompanied by increased energy and reduced tension. If the five-minute walk doesn't affect your urge, you might try ten minutes—or you might get by with two minutes, or even just some stretching wherever you are. Your aim will be to find out how your appetite and your moods react to moderate exercise.

In addition to studying the effects of moderate exercise on your moods, it is useful to know the effects of more demanding exercise. If you are used to doing forty-five minutes of aerobics, or running five miles, you should become familiar with exactly how these levels of physical activity change your mood. (Experienced exercisers are often very aware of this.) Measuring your energy and tension before and after such activities can be very enlightening. But here, it is important to pay attention to how you feel an hour or two later, in addition to immediately afterward. You may find that energy is decreased from vigorous physical activity, but after you recover a bit you have a burst of energy that lasts for some time.

Based on research now being conducted on the positive mood effects of resistance exercise (for example, weight lifting), you might also want to vary the amount of this kind of exercise, and pay attention to energy and tension changes immediately after it as well as some time later. It is likely that muscle tension is an important part of psychological tension, so resistance exercise, which stresses and relaxes various muscles, could have a very positive effect on anxiety, in addition to the natural energy surge it gives you.

Relaxation Techniques

Throughout this book we have seen that by increasing your energy, reducing your tension, or both, you can change a bad mood. We have seen that exercise increases energy and also reduces tension, making exercise a sure bet. But other methods of tension reduction are well known and effective. Although many are familiar with relaxation techniques—or stress management activities, as they are sometimes known—not many use them. Part of the reason for this, I am convinced, is that they have not sufficiently recognized the positive effects these methods have in regulating mood. Nor have the long-term effects on eating and exercise of these practices been recognized. Another reason for not using these techniques is that they require practice before their benefits can be fully realized.

Unlike the immediate effects of a ten-minute brisk walk, meditation and other similar approaches take time to learn. They can be very effective methods of reducing tension, but they usually cannot be used just once with an expectation of much success.

Stress management activities work in various ways. To oversimplify, I believe that muscle relaxation and massage reduce muscle tension directly, and usually this has a constructive effect on thoughts, which tend to correspond in positive or negative ways to our body tension. Many forms of meditation and visualization that involve focused attention, on the other hand, enable the proficient user to control his or her tension-inducing thoughts, and this in turn reduces tense arousal throughout the body. Systems like yoga, tai chi, and other forms of meditative exercise that involve the body and the mind simultaneously influence both muscle tension and cognitive systems at the same time. Learning to control both your thoughts and your muscle tension is quite feasible, but it takes practice. You wouldn't expect to play proficient tennis after one lesson, and something similar is true of controlling your thoughts in meditation or learning to relax your muscles.

Tension reduction can have a remarkable effect on unnecessary eating. You can see one clear indication of this by practicing meditation before dinner or other meals. You will still experience hunger, but probably not as urgently. You will also eat more slowly and enjoy the food more. If the meditation was effective and you feel calm from it, eating will be a quiet, pleasurable experience with no sense of rushing. And you will eat less.

Many books can help you become proficient with these techniques for tension reduction. For example, Herbert Benson, the Harvard Medical School physician who pioneered research on simple methods of meditation, argues in his book *The Relaxation Response* that there are four basic components necessary to bring forth this form of relaxation, which he characterizes as the opposite of the fight-or-flight response: a quiet environment, a mental device to focus your thoughts (like a sound, word, or phrase repeated silently), a passive attitude (not pursuing thoughts that come to consciousness, but simply returning to the repetition of the mental device), and a comfortable position (no undue muscular tension).[5]

The mental device represents a kind of control of your thoughts. When you are concentrating on a pleasant word or phrase, you are not thinking about your problems or other anxiety-inducing matters. This is variously described by different experts on stress management as mindfulness, living in the moment, visualization of pleasant scenes, or other forms of focused attention. Some practitioners argue that the focus of attention should be positive phrases about yourself, or so-called self-affirmations. All these methods, however, enable you to focus your attention away from thoughts that generate anxiety and toward something that is positive or neutral.

Use Benson's technique or any other good one that you might choose, and assess your tension before and after each session (using a five- or seven-point scale). Pay attention to how you feel an hour or two afterward, as well. You might want to practice your stress management technique before a mealtime to determine whether it makes you eat less food in a more relaxed state. It will be invaluable for you to understand how your moods affect your eating.

Although reducing tension usually is the major effect of meditation and other forms of stress management, you will also notice that your energy increases, especially if the relaxation technique is practiced during an otherwise high-energy time of day. For example, in his book *Breathing: The Master Key to Self-Healing,* the well-known naturalistic physician Andrew Weil argues that certain breathing exercises can relax tension, while others can increase energy.[6] Breathing exercises are basic elements of many forms of stress management, since rapid and shallow respiration characterizes tension, and controlled breathing can regulate this function. If we make ourselves breathe with a pattern that is characteristic of relaxation, it will calm us down. Weil also observes that in his experience various urges are effectively eliminated by these exercises, and this is to be expected if they reduce tension and increase energy. You might wish to try two breathing techniques (see endnote for procedure) on a number of occasions, and rate your feelings of energy and tension before and after.[7] Also notice your reactions to food after these exercises.

Still another technique combines the energy-enhancing effects of a short brisk walk with a kind of meditation. Originated by media pundit T George Harris, this is a relaxation technique that could be particularly effective if you feel like taking a walk but you don't feel like sitting and meditating.[8] With this technique, while you walk you count each time one foot hits the ground. Or you may repeat your favorite song in rhythm with your steps. More recently, working with Benedictine monks, Harris found that repeating a meaningful prayer phrase combines prayerfulness with exercise and mental control.[9] If you try this exercise, rate your energy and tension before and after each time you do it, also noting your reactions to food.

Cognitive Override

In managing both urges to eat and reluctance to exercise, you can use your mind effectively by employing what I call cognitive override, which involves a kind of mental control. Let us consider how this works.

When you have done all, or even some, of the self-studies suggested in this chapter, you will know a lot about your moods. You will recognize how a tense tired state can make you break a diet, even when you are firmly resolved not to do that. And you will realize the way that natural cycles of low energy make exercise especially unappealing at certain times. But you will also gain knowledge from your self-studies about what you can do to overcome these moods. They will give you the tools to manage your mood.

We have seen that there are many ways of effectively dealing with tense tiredness: moderate exercise, a nap, a small amount of nutrition, muscle relaxation, recognizing a bad time of day and avoiding negative thoughts at that time. These and many other ways are helpful if you realize that the problem is low energy and high tension. It is here that cognitive override can be beneficial. Whether you call it the power of thought, or just gritting your teeth and exercising because you know it will have a positive effect, what cognitive override does is to use your knowledge to resist food urges or, if necessary, make you exercise when you don't want to.[10]

When an urge to break your diet hits and all you can think about is your favorite good-tasting food, cognitive override involves remembering what you have learned about the way tense tiredness inflames such urges and what can be done to counteract this negative state. Unlike the ways you have tried to avoid such urges before and failed, with cognitive override you will find it easier because the knowledge you have gained from self-studies has given you a way to facilitate control. For example, if you realize that the low energy you are feeling comes from sitting around too much, you will know from personal experience that a little exercise may do the trick. Or, if you recognize tense tiredness for what causes it, you may realize that you haven't slept enough lately, and perhaps a nap now and a resolve to sleep more in the future are what you need. Or, from your self-study you may think about what time of day it is, and, if this is one of your low periods, one possibility is simply to avoid eating for a little while until this hour passes. It's easier to do if you know that the time you have to wait is limited, and if you know that your urge may soon pass in the same way that your energy naturally varies up and down. In each of these cases, and many more, your knowledge about your moods gives you information that you can use to override the insistent urges.

If you feel tense and tired, one of your first options is to remember your experience with moderate exercise and to use a short brisk walk or some other physical activity intentionally to raise your energy and reduce your appetite. Although beginning to exercise may be difficult, if you have done the self-study on how exercise affects your moods, you will know that even a small amount of exercise will raise your energy and reduce your urge, and you will know how physical activity probably will rev up your body just enough so that more exercise becomes naturally appealing. This will enable you to override your negative inclinations.

Another possibility is that you might practice a relaxation method when the urge hits. If you have done the self-study and observed how relaxation techniques reduce your tension, you will be motivated to use that approach. It will be inviting and you will look forward to it because you will have experienced its reinforcing effects. Again, the knowledge gained from your self-studies will help you to exert cognitive override.

Recognizing mild tense tiredness and its implications is really the secret. When you know all about this state you will realize that you should deal with it as soon as it appears, before it becomes too strong to control. As before, your knowledge of your moods from self-study, together with your knowledge of ways of counteracting tense tiredness, will give you this information. Forewarned, you will realize that your resources are flagging and that if you let yourself go without repairing the deficit, it will only get worse.

From your self-studies of stress, you will know in advance what to expect when you are experiencing a stressful period and what your actual experience of stress feels like. You will realize why fast foods and snacks become more attractive during stress, and if your problem is flagging energy and increased tension, you will have some tools for dealing with these feelings so you can avoid a busted diet.

Feelings of depression, which in the past have driven you to eat, will become less mysterious once you have studied yourself. Depressing thoughts about yourself and the future will be recognized as coming in part from natural reactions of reduced energy and the consequent vulnerability to increased tension. Rather than entertaining thoughts that your life is worthless, which send you into an eating binge, you will understand that your thoughts are strongly influenced by natural mood processes, and this will give you an amount of control.

When exercise and relaxation methods are called for, inevitably you will experience countervailing thoughts that you just don't want to exercise now, or it's just too much effort to do your relaxation exercises. You will want to eat and relax instead. But your knowledge gained from self-study will make you an expert on yourself so that you can activate your power of self-control. What you are doing in all these cases is using your knowledge—your mind—to override the negative urges fostered by powerful moods. And you can do this because you have the undeniable evidence from your own experience.

Appendix

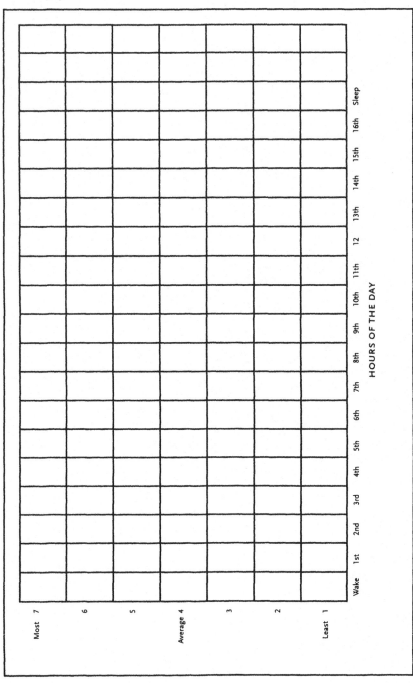

At this moment, how energetic, vigorous, and full of pep do I feel? (Mark box with an O)

1   2   3   4   5   6   7

least   average   most

At this moment, how tense, jittery, and intense do I feel? (Mark box with an X)

1   2   3   4   5   6   7

least   average   most

Mark a U when you have the urge to eat.

Notes

Chapter 1   Mood, Self-Regulation, and Overeating

1. I have outlined the scientific evidence for these assertions in my two books, *The biopyschology of mood and arousal* (1989) and *The origin of everyday moods* (1996), both published by Oxford University Press.

2. Quite a few other researchers are actively studying this hot topic. For example, see the following analyses J. J. Gross, Emotion regulation: Past, present, future, *Cognition and Emotion* 13 (1999): 551–73; R. J. Larsen, Toward a science of mood regulation, *Psychological Inquiry* 11 (2000): 129–41; B. Parkinson and P. Totterdell, Classifying affect-regulation strategies, *Cognition and Emotion* 13 (1999): 277–303; D. M. Tice and E. Bratslavsky, Giving in to feel good: The place of emotion regulation in the context of general self-control, *Psychological Inquiry* 11 (2000): 149–59.

3. The most complete scientific report of our findings can be found in R. E. Thayer, J. R. Newman, and T. M. McClain, The self-regulation of mood: Strategies for changing a bad mood, raising energy, and reducing tension, *Journal of Personality and Social Psychology* 67 (1994): 910–25. This research has since generated a great deal of interest among psychologists.

4. Shelly Taylor and her colleagues at the University of California, Los Angeles, describe a characteristic, especially of women, to "tend and befriend," which they see as being linked to various neural and hormonal systems. See Chapter 8 in this book, *Calm energy;* S. E. Taylor,

L. C. Klein, B. P. Lewis, T. L. Gruenewald, R. A. R Gurung, and J. A. Updegraff, Biobehavioral responses to stress in females: Tend-and-befriend, not fight-or-flight, *Psychological Review* 107 (2000): 411–29.

5. Thayer, Newman, and McClain, "Self-regulation of mood."

6. Ibid. See also Roper poll data discussed in Chapter 2.

7. R. E. Thayer, Energy, tiredness and tension effects of a sugar snack versus moderate exercise, *Journal of Personality and Social Psychology* 52 (1987a): 119–25.

8. Decades of behavioral research on learning show that reinforcers occurring immediately after a behavior control that behavior, even if different reactions occur later.

9. R. M. Ganley, Emotion and eating in obesity: A review of the literature, *International Journal of Eating Disorders* 8 (1989): 342–61

10. Ganley makes a good case for emotional eating as a cause of obesity; some reviews support his viewpoint and others take slightly different perspectives, based mainly on methodological limitations. See E. Abramson, *Emotional eating* (New York: Lexington Books, 1993); D. B. Allison and S. Heshka, Emotion and eating in obesity? A critical analysis, *International Journal of Eating Disorders* 13 (1993): 289–95; L. Christensen, Effects of eating behavior on mood: A review of the literature, *International Journal of Eating Disorders* 14 (1993): 171–83; M. S. Faith, D. B. Allison, and A. Geliebter, Emotional eating and obesity: Theoretical considerations and practical recommendations, in *Overweight and weight management*, ed. S. Dalton (Gaithersburg, Md.: Aspen Publishers, 1997); G. G. Greeno and R. R. Wing, Stress-induced eating, *Psychological Bulletin* 115 (1994): 444–64.

11. We know from careful psychometric studies that alertness and energy are closely related (R. E. Thayer, Factor analytic and reliability studies on the Activation-Deactivation Adjective Check List, *Psychological Reports* 42 [1978a]: 747–56).

12. Thayer, Energy, tiredness, and tension effects of a sugar snack.

13. This theory was first proposed in Thayer, Energy, tiredness, and tension effects of a sugar snack.

14. This is essentially an evolutionary argument. The ancestral bases of these reactions extend back at least several million years, probably developing through the process of natural selection.

15. D. B. Herzog, K. M. Nussbaum, and A. K. Marmor, Comorbidity and

outcome in eating disorders, *The Psychiatric Clinics of North America* 19 (1996): 843–59.

16. These arguments are developed further in Thayer, *Origin of everyday moods.*

17. This relationship is not proved, but it is supported by much anecdotal evidence.

18. In one interesting study showing how starchy foods stimulate snacking, obese boys were fed either high starchy foods (for example, instant oatmeal with a high glycemic index) or low starchy foods (for example, vegetable omelet and fruit), but with the same energy content and palatability. Those boys who ate the high starchy food chose to eat 81 percent more snacks in the next five hours than those fed the low starchy food (D. S. Ludwig, et al., High glycemic index foods, overeating, and obesity, *Pediatrics,* 103 [1999]: E26).

19. R. F. Baumeister, T. F. Heatherton, and D. M. Tice, *Losing control: How and why people fail at self-regulation* (San Diego, Calif.: Academic Press, 1994).

20. R. E. Thayer, D. P. Peters, P. J. Takahashi, and A. M. Birkhead-Flight, Mood and behavior (smoking and sugar snacking) following moderate exercise: A partial test of self-regulation theory, *Personality and Individual Differences* 14 (1993): 97–104.

Chapter 2   Living in a Stressful World: Mood and Overweight

1. For example, in a Princeton Survey Research Associates poll (ending date: January 1999), 41 percent of adult women reported being overweight, and in a Hart and Teeter Research Companies poll (ending date: June 21, 1998), 46 percent of adults and 50 percent of women reported being overweight. When "overweight" is broken down into differing amounts, almost two-thirds indicate overweight. (For example, a Hart and Teeter Research Companies poll, ending date: June 25, 1996, showed 63 percent of adults and 68 percent of women indicating overweight.) In a Gallup poll taken in 1989 (ending date: September 15), however, 33 percent of adults described themselves as overweight, and a Harris poll taken in 1980 (ending date: December 6) found that 36 percent described themselves as overweight. Thus, self-descriptions of overweight have been increasing in recent years.

These poll data and other data that follow can be found through the POLL database of the Roper Center at the University of Connecticut.

2. Conducted by the Center for Disease Control and Prevention and state health departments, this cross-sectional telephone survey of more than 100,000 participants eighteen years or older is likely to have underestimated the amount of obesity because self-estimates tend to underestimate height and weight, and also those without telephones, unreachable through this survey, are likely to have higher weight (A. H. Mokdad, et al., The spread of the obesity epidemic in the United States, 1991–1998, *Journal of the American Medical Association*, 282 [1999]: 1519–22). More accurate estimates based on measures taken by health professionals in the National Health and Nutrition Examinations Surveys (see below) showed one-third greater degrees of obesity.

3. Body image: An in-depth look at how we see ourselves, *Psychology Today*, January/February 1997.

4. In a Harris poll (ending date: July 16, 1995), 63 percent of American adults said that being substantially overweight is because of the genes you inherit. These perceptions have been changing as the public becomes more familiar with genetic research. In a Roper poll taken in 1979 (ending date: September 29), only 36 percent said that overweight is due to heredity.

5. G. A. Bray, B. York, and J. Delany, A survey of the opinions of obesity experts on the causes and treatment of obesity, *American Journal of Clinical Nutrition* 55 (1992): 151–54S.

6. For example, a recent British study showed that, among women with overweight or obese twin sisters, higher levels of physical activity were associated with a 3.96–kilogram (nearly 9–pound) lower total body fat (K. Samparas, et al., Genetic and environmental influences on total-body and central abdominal fat: The effect of physical activity in female twins, *Annals of Internal Medicine*, 130 [1999]: 873–82).

7. G. Taubes, As obesity rates rise, experts struggle to explain why, *Science* 280 (1998): 1367–68. See also K. M. Flegal, M. D. Carroll, R. J. Kuczmarski, and C. L. Johnson, Overweight and obesity in the United States: Prevalence and trends, 1960–1994, *International Journal of Obesity Research Relating to Metabolic Disorders* 22 (1998): 39–47.

Also see a number of articles in the *Journal of the American Medical Association*'s special issue on obesity: 282 (October 27, 1999).

8. On obesity being a worldwide trend, especially in Western societies, see Taubes, As obesity rates rise.

9. Many experts recommend BMIs no greater than 25, although there is disagreement about how important those between twenty-six and twenty-seven are. There is some consensus that BMIs over thirty increase the risk of death (I. Wickelgren, Obesity: How big a problem? *Science* 280 [1998]: 1364–67).

10. The most reliable data indicating this change in body weight come from National Health and Nutrition Examination Surveys (NHANES) between 1960 and 1994. These include both home interviews and physical examinations in specially equipped mobile examination centers.

11. H. B. Hubert, M. Feinleib, P. M. McNamara, and W. P. Castelli, Obesity as an independent risk factor for cardiovascular disease: A 26–year follow-up of participants in the Framingham Heart Study, *Circulation* 67 (1983): 968–77.

12. J. E. Manson, et al., Body weight and mortality among women, *New England Journal of Medicine* 333 (1995): 677–85.

13. J. Stevens, J. Cai, E. R. Pamuk, D. F. Williamson, M. J. Thun, and J. L. Wood, The effect of age on the association between body-mass index and mortality, *New England Journal of Medicine* 338 (1998): 1–7.

14. A. Must, et al., The disease burden associated with overweight and obesity, *Journal of the American Medical Association* 282 (1999): 1523–29.

15. In recent research with over 21,000 men thirty to eighty-three years of age, Blair and his colleagues concluded, "The health benefits of leanness are limited to fit men, and being fit may reduce the hazards of obesity" (C. D. Lee, S. N. Blair, and A. S. Jackson, Cardiorespiratory fitness, body composition, and all-cause and cardiovascular disease mortality in men, *American Journal of Clinical Nutrition* 69 [1999]: 373–80).

16. These included the following polls and results: Louis Harris and Associates (ending date: November 8, 1983): 16 percent said they were under stress almost every day; Harris (ending date: November 15, 1984): 13 percent; Harris (ending date: September 1985): 8 percent;

Harris (ending date: November 26, 1985): 14 percent; Harris (ending date: November 25, 1987): 17 percent; Harris, (ending date: November 23, 1988): 18 percent; and Harris (ending date: December 13, 1989): 15 percent.

17. Louis Harris and Associates (ending date: November 29, 1990): 16 percent said they were under stress almost every day; Princeton Survey Research (ending date: February 10, 1991): 22 percent; Harris (ending date: December 5, 1991): 18 percent; Princeton (ending date: December 4, 1992): 17 percent; Princeton (ending date: November 23, 1993): 19 percent; Princeton (ending date: August 4, 1994): 14 percent; and Princeton (ending date November 15, 1994): 21 percent. Other polls asking slightly different questions nonetheless showed similar results. For example, in 1990 a Research and Forcasts poll (ending date: January 7) found that 50 percent of respondents were more stressed compared to five years earlier. In 1991 63 percent of respondents to a Roper poll (ending date: January 30) said they were more stressed compared to their parents. In 1994 a Gallup poll (ending date: November 4) found that 40 percent of respondents frequently experience stress in their daily life. And in 1997 a Princeton survey found that 73 percent felt the average person is more stressed than 20 years ago. These changing levels of stress do not apply only to older adults. In a 1999 annual survey of over 360,000 college freshmen, 30.2 percent said that they frequently feel overwhelmed by all they have to do, but in 1985 only 16 percent answered this way (Reuters, January 24, 2000). It is obvious that stress is increasing throughout the society.

18. In addition to women reporting more stress than men in many polls on everyday stress in which a breakdown was made, women may have a more realistic perception of stress than men. For example, in a 1997 Princeton Survey Research poll (ending date: July 9), 79 percent of women thought the average person was under more stress than twenty or thirty years ago, compared with only 68 percent of men. Both percentages of perceived stress are very high, of course, but more women see the problem as being greater than men do, and this perception alone could be the reason for increased self-regulation with food.

19. A. Toffler, *Future shock* (New York: Random House, 1970).

20. J. Glick, *Faster: The acceleration of just about everything* (New York: Pantheon Books, 1999). Jacket copy.

21. Gordon S. Black Corporation poll (ending date: February 1987).

22. Roper Organization poll (ending date: December 3, 1994).

23. K.R.C. Research and Consulting poll (ending date: November 7, 1995).

24. Personal business, *Atlanta Journal and Constitution*, July 22, 1996.

25. National Public Radio special featuring Leah Fisher and others, July 6, 1998.

26. Working on stress, *USA Today*, May 5, 1998.

27. Hectic workplace, *Miami Herald*, September 7, 1998.

28. A *Washington Post* poll of adults in 1997 (ending date: September 14) found in response to the question, "How many hours per week do you work?" that the average was 44 hours, while in two Gallup Organization polls conducted in 1989 (ending dates: December 21), men averaged 42.8 hours and women, 36.7 hours.

29. Temps take on a full-time role, *Los Angeles Times*, May 29, 1999.

30. A growing workplace threat, *The Kansas City Star*, January 31, 1999.

31. Workplace absenteeism, *St. Louis Post Dispatch*, October 25, 1998.

32. Gallup Organization poll (ending date: February 1998).

33. *Washington Post* poll (ending date: September 14, 1997).

34. Princeton Survey Research Associates poll (ending date: July 9, 1997). And 79 percent of women thought there was more stress compared to 68 percent of men. Once again, this is evidence that women are under more stress.

35. Gordon S. Black Corporation polls (ending date: February 1987 [married respondents], 13 percent; ending date: February 1987 [single, divorced, widowed], 15 percent; ending date: July 7, 1984, 15 percent.)

36. Internet boosts productivity but adds stress, *USA Today*, March 18, 1988.

37. Wirtlin Group poll (ending date: April 9, 1993).

38. Research and Forecasts poll (ending date: January 7, 1990).

39. R. E. Thayer, J. R. Newman, and T. M. McClain, The self-regulation of mood: Strategies for changing a bad mood, raising energy, and reducing tension, *Journal of Personality and Social Psychology* 67 (1994): 910–25.

40. In 1987 a Roper poll (ending date: September 26) showed that 14 percent often exercised as a way of dealing with stress, and 22 per-

cent sometimes exercised. But by 1994, 42 percent in a Gallup poll (ending date: January 30) indicated that they exercised or walked to relieve stress.

41. Roper Organization (ending date: August 12, 1989).

42. A kind of confirmation for these findings as applied to wider health factors came from a study of over 19,000 adults throughout the United States, which concluded that social relationships have a beneficial effect on several behaviors that directly or indirectly affect the risk of cardiovascular disease (E. S. Ford, I. B. Ahluwalia, and D. A. Galuski, Social relationships and cardiovascular disease risk factors: Findings from the third national health and nutrition examination survey, *Preventive Medicine* 30 [2000]: 83–92).

43. A Roper poll (ending date: August 12, 1989) found that 15 percent of women often work on a hobby when stressed and 28 percent sometimes do (16 percent and 29 percent of men).

44. Roper Organization poll (ending date: August 12, 1989).

45. In a Roper poll (ending date: August 12, 1989), 38 percent of women reported that they often watch TV as a way of dealing with stress, and 39 percent said they watch it sometimes for this purpose. The comparable figures for men were 36 percent often and 37 percent sometimes.

46. S. R. Maddi, The personality construct of hardiness: I. Effects on experiencing, coping, and strain, *Consulting Psychology Journal: Practice and Research* 51 (1999): 83–94.

47. L. N. Robins, et al., Lifetime prevalence of specific psychiatric disorders in three sites, *Archives of General Psychiatry* 41 (1984): 949–58; L. N. Robins, B. Z. Locke, and D. A. Regier, An overview of psychiatric disorders in America, *Psychiatric disorder in America: The epidemiologic catchment area study*, ed. L. N. Robins and D. A. Regier (New York: Free Press, 1991).

48. R. C. Kessler, et al., Lifetime and 12–month prevalence of DSM-III-R psychiatric disorders in the United States, *Archives of General Psychiatry* 51 (1994): 8–19. These two National Institute of Mental Health and congressionally mandated studies have been the main sources of data in the United States on the prevalence of psychiatric disorders. No more recent study of this magnitude has been conducted, but additional data are being gathered. In a follow-up study of the relationship

between job stress and depression, 904 respondents working in occupations with high psychologic strain showed greater prevalence of major depressive episodes, depressive syndrome, and dysphoria. This study provides good evidence of a link between job stress and depression (H. Mausner-Dorsch and W. W. Eaton, Psychosocial work environment and depression: Epidemiologic assessment of the demand-control model, *American Journal of Public Health* 90 [2000]: 1765–70).

49. R. M. Hirschfeld, et al., The National Depressive and Manic-Depressive Association consensus statement on the undertreatment of depression, *Journal of the American Medical Association* 277 (1997): 333–340.

50. See *Feelings: Our vital signs*, a very readable description of the significance of these feelings by psychiatrist Willard Gaylin (New York: Ballantine, 1979).

51. These two government studies differed somewhat in their sampling techniques and ways of questioning respondents, but in my view, if anything, these differences could have minimized the growth in depression and related disorders that was observed. For example, the first study focused on urban areas, while the second one took a more representative sample of Americans. Because psychiatric disorders tend to be greater in urban areas, the first study may have slightly overestimated the prevalence of psychiatric disorders for Americans at that time, and therefore there could be even greater increases in depression in this ten-year period than I have indicated. In addition to these authoritative government studies, two recent meta-analyses comparing the effects obtained in a number of other studies showed the presence of substantially higher levels of anxiety in recent decades. Both college student and child samples evidenced increases in anxiety of almost a full standard deviation between 1952 and 1993. J. M. Twenge, The age of anxiety?: The birth cohort change in anxiety and neuroticism, 1952–1993, *Journal of Personality and Social Psychology* 79 (2000): 1007–21.

52. Reuters, May 17, 2000; K. Harby, Childhood psychiatric emergencies on the rise.

53. K. J. Kelleher, T. K. McInerny, W. P. Gardner, G. E. Childs, and R. C. Wasserman, Increasing identification of psychosocial problems: 1979–1996, *Pediatrics* 105 (2000): 1313–21.

54. *Los Angeles Times* (ending date: April 6, 1989).
55. Wirthlin Group (ending date: January 1996).
56. Princeton Survey Research Associates (ending date: January 1999).
57. As one study by the Department of Health and Human Services, Public Health Service, (July 9, 1996) indicated, the proportion of adults with affective disorders who are not treated is almost three times greater than the proportion that is treated.

Chapter 3   How Are Exercise and Mood Related?

1. At the time of this writing, MEDLINE yields 33,456 scientific articles with *exercise* in the title, and from a sample of them it appears that exercise shows favorable effects in most of this research.
2. D. S. Lauderdale, et al., Familial determinants of moderate and intense physical activity: A twin study, *Medicine and Science in Sports and Exercise* 29 (1997): 1062–68.
3. Science file, Stone age aerobics, *Los Angeles Times*, January 27, 1997; L. Cordain, R. W. Gotshall, and S. B. Eaton, Evolutionary aspects of exercise, *World Review of Nutrition and Dietetics* 81 (1997): 49–60.
4. One authoritative review sets an optimal type of physical activity to enhance health at 50 percent of an individual's maximal oxygen intake, sustained for one hour three to five times per week (R. J. Shephard, What is the optimal type of physical activity to enhance health? *British Journal of Sports Medicine* 31 [1997]: 277–84).
5. G. A. Rose and R. T. Williams, Metabolic studies of large and small eaters, *British Journal of Nutrition* 15 (1961): 1–9.
6. J. A. Levine, N. L. Eberhardt, and M. D. Jensen, Role of nonexercise activity thermogenesis in resistance to fat gain in humans, *Science* 283 (1999): 212–14.
7. You can begin to see the complexity of the energy-in/energy-out relationship from research that shows that even so small an expenditure of energy as gum chewing raises metabolism—20 percent in one report (J. Levine, P. Baukol, and I. Pavlidis, The energy expended in chewing gum, *New England Journal of Medicine* 341 [1999]: 2100).
8. For a consideration of the general theoretical issues, see J. E. Blundell and N. A. King, Effects of exercise on appetite control: Loose coupling between energy expenditure and energy intake, *International Journal of Obesity* 22 (1998): S22–29.

9. For a review of the literature, see N. A. King, A. Tremblay, and J. E. Blundell, Effects of exercise on appetite control: Implications for energy balance, *Medicine and Science in Sports and Exercise* 29 (1996): 1076–89.

10. J. Mayer, N. B. Marshall, J. J. Vitale, J. H. Christensen, M. B. Mashayekhi, and F. J. Stare, Exercise, food intake and body weight in normal rats and genetically obese adult mice, *American Journal of Physiology* 177 (1954): 544–48.

11. The evidence here is unclear. It is curious, but apparently the federal government, including the President's Council on Physical Fitness, keeps no ongoing statistics about how much Americans exercise. Two researchers who study activity patterns argue that in the 1990s "the love affair Americans have with fitness may be on the decline. Many weekend athletes have hung up their shoes, according to the National Center for Health Statistics data" (J. P. Robinson and G. Godbey, *Time for life: The surprising ways Americans use their time* [University Park: Pennsylvania State University Press, 1997], p. 181). However, the Sporting Goods Manufacturers Association, which keeps track of exercise equipment sales, provided me with statistics indicating that there has been a steady trend toward increasing purchases over the past decade. Nevertheless, it may be true that people are buying more exercise equipment but not using it.

12. Tracking reported sleep length over the past fifteen years is a good indication that people feel they have less time. This is because when there is too little time, sleep is one of the first things to go. Public opinion polls taken from national samples show that today people are sleeping less than seven hours a night, but ten years ago they were sleeping between seven and eight hours a night. This difference is small but significant. Moreover, evidence indicates that this speeding up of American society as reflected in lessened sleep time has been occurring for quite a while. For example, adults responded to the question of how many hours a night they sleep in a 1996 Gallup poll with the reported average of 6.9 hours (ending date: July 21); another 1996 Gallup poll indicated 6.8 hours. Responses of adults to a 1994 Princeton Survey Research poll showed 7.0 hours (ending date: November 15). But in 1989, a Harris poll clocked usual sleeping time at 7.3 hours (ending date: December 13), and a Harris poll

in 1984 found an average of 7.4 hours (ending date: March 15).
Going back to 1947, a Gallup poll found that adults slept 8.1 hours
(ending date: April 2). There are variations over the years in the
results of the many polls that have asked about sleeping time, but the
trend toward decreasing sleep is unmistakable. See also J. B. Maas,
Power sleep (New York: Villard, 1998).

13. Although not directly applicable to Mary, serious depression has lots
of signs. The whole body announces the condition—everything from
slumped shoulders and slow movement to bowed head and facial
expressions that are empty of vigor. Then, of course, there are the
constant expressions of sadness and negative thinking about everything from yourself to the future. Or, there is overtly self-destructive
behavior. These signs of serious depression are relatively easy to spot.
Moderate depression of the kind that Mary experienced, on the other
hand, is a more subtle condition. But in this moderate state you can
see some of the same characteristics evident in serious depression,
and Mary experienced these in lesser degrees.

14. An important question about depression concerns whether reduced
energy is the most important element of this condition or whether
the most important elements involve well-known associated cognitions and attributions such as low life satisfaction, lack of perception
of control, low self-esteem, and poor expectancies. In other words, is
low energy the best defining characteristic of depression, or do cognitive variables best define this negative state? A particularly impressive demonstration of the fundamental importance of energetic
arousal in depression as opposed to related cognitions comes from a
study by L. Christensen and K. Duncan and a subsequent re-analysis
of that data (Larry Christensen, personal communication, 2000). In
this research, energetic arousal—that is, low energy—correctly predicted 93 percent of depressed subjects with negative cognitions held
constant, but when measures of energetic arousal were held constant,
depression was less predictable from cognitive variables. This suggests
that, in the depressed condition, low energy produces negative cognitions rather than negative cognitions producing low energy (L. Christensen and K. Duncan, Distinguishing depressed from nondepressed
individuals using energy and psychosocial variables, *Journal of Consulting and Clinical Psychology* 63 [1995]: 495–98).

15. Exercise scientist William Morgan from the University of Wisconsin
    reviewed the extensive literature on the relationship between exer-
    cise and depression and, although cautious, as scientists usually are,
    he concluded that there is compelling evidence that exercise is associ-
    ated with decreased levels of mild to moderate depression. One of
    the problems with the scientific literature in this area that prevents
    him from being even more emphatic is the absence of clear proof of
    cause and effect is a problem that arises from correlational studies.
    See W. P. Morgan, Physical activity, fitness and depression, in *Physical
    activity, fitness, and health: International proceedings and consensus state-
    ment*, ed. C. Bouchard, R. J. Shephard, and T. Stephens (Champaign,
    Ill.: Human Kenetics Publishers, 1994), 851–67. Also see a more
    recent review that draws similar conclusions: D. Scully, J. Kremer, M.
    M. Meade, R. Graham, and K. Dudgeon, Physical exercise and psy-
    chological well being: A critical review, *British Journal of Sports Medi-
    cine* 32 (1998): 111–20.
16. R. B. Bassin, The relationship of exercise, self-reported depression
    and activation level, Master's thesis, California State University, Long
    Beach, 1989.
17. W. Gaylin, *Feelings: Our Vital Signs* (New York: Ballantine, 1979).
18. I reviewed and cited a number of studies indicating the relationship
    between moderate exercise and energy enhancement in my earlier
    two books, *The biopsychology of mood and arousal* (1989) and *The origin
    of everyday moods* (1996), both published by Oxford University Press.
    New studies continue to provide evidence for this relationship. For
    example, A. K. Tate and S. J. Petruzzello studied twenty students who
    engaged in thirty minutes of cycling on an exercise bike in separate
    conditions at 55 percent VO_2 max (corresponding to light exercise)
    and 70 percent VO_2 max (perceived exertion between somewhat
    hard and hard). These were regular exercisers who worked out very
    hard 4.2 times a week, on average. Subjective energy significantly
    increased during the exercise in both conditions, and the elevated
    energy continued for the thirty minutes after the exercise during
    which measurements were taken (A. K. Tate, and S. J. Petruzzello,
    Varying the intensity of acute exercise: Implications for changes in
    affect, *Journal of Sports Medicine and Physical Fitness* 35 [1995]:
    295–302).

19. R. E. Thayer, Energy, tiredness, and tension effects of a sugar snack versus moderate exercise, *Journal of Personality and Social Psychology* 52 (1987a): 119–25.

20. D. H. Saklofske and his associates later replicated these findings, and similar results have now been obtained in other research as well (D. H. Saklofske, G. C. Blomme, and I. W. Kelly, The effect of exercise and relaxation on energetic and tense arousal, *Personality and Individual Differences* 13 [1992]: 623–25). Results consistent with these were also found in several naturalistic and laboratory studies using ten- to fifteen-minute walks (for example, P. Ekkekakis, E. E. Hall, L. M. Van Landuyt, and S. J. Petruzzello, Walking in (affective) circles: Can short walks enhance affect? *Journal of Behavioral Medicine* 23 [2000]: 245–75).

21. L. Gauvin, W. J. Rejeski, and J. L. Norris, A naturalistic study of the impact of acute physical activity on feeling states and affect in women, *Health Psychology* 15 (1996): 391–97.

22. G. Brown, *The energy of life* (New York: Free Press, 2000).

23. See Chapter 8 for further discussion of this matter. Also, a variety of other specific physiological and psychological bases for mood change from exercise in addition to those already mentioned above have been hypothesized (for example, see the brief listing in S. Weyerer and B. Kupfer, Physical exercise and psychological health, *Sports Medicine* 17 [1994]: 108–16). Also note some interesting research on lateralized shifts in brain activation (S. J. Petruzzello and D. M. Landers, State anxiety reduction and exercise: Does hemispheric activation reflect such changes? *Medicine Science in Sports and Exercise* 26 [1994]: 1028–35).

24. See P. Ekkekakis and S. J. Petruzzello, Acute aerobic exercise and affect: Current status, problems, and prospects regarding dose-response, *Sports Medicine* 28 (1999): 337–74; L. Gauvin and J. C. Spence, Physical activity and psychological well-being: Knowledge base, current issues, and caveats, *Nutrition Reviews* 54 (1996): S53–65; S. J. Petruzzello, D. M. Landers, B. D. Hatfield, K. A. Kubitz, and W. Salazar, A meta-analysis on the anxiety-reducing effects of acute and chronic exercise, *Sports Medicine* 11 (1991): 143–82; and R. R. Yeung, The acute effects of exercise on mood states, *Journal of psychosomatic research* 40 (1996): 123–41.

25. N. P. Pronk, S. F. Crouse, and J. J. Rohack, Maximal exercise and acute mood response in women, *Physiology and Behavior* 57 (1995): 1–4.

26. A. Steptoe and S. Cox, Acute effects of aerobic exercise on mood, *Health Psychology* 7 (1988): 329–40.

27. P. Ekkekakis, E. E. Hall, and S. J. Petruzzello, however, make the excellent point that this apparent increase in anxiety may be related to measurement error that occurs when using the State-Trait Anxiety Questionnaire (STAI; C. D. Spielberger, *Manual for the State-Trait Anxiety Inventory* (form Y) [Palo Alto, Calif.: Consulting Psychologists Press, 1983]), a test that has been used by many exercise scientists to assess anxiety reactions. They provide empirical results in two experiments to show that the STAI is actually a multidimensional test that measures different kinds of anxiety reactions, and they show further that the assumed increase in anxiety immediately following exercise is better represented as both increased activation and effort-related tension. This is a "tense-energy" response, to use the term employed in this book (P. Ekkekakis, E. E. Hall, and S. J. Petruzzello, Measuring state anxiety in the context of acute exercise using the State Anxiety Inventory: An attempt to resolve the brouhaha, *Journal of Sport and Exercise Psychology* 21 [1999]: 205–29).

28. J. S. Raglin and M. Wilson, State anxiety following 20 minutes of bicycle ergometric exercise at selected intensities, *International Journal of Sports Medicine* 17 (1996): 467–71. See also P. J. O'Connor, S. J. Petruzzello, K. A. Kubitz, and T. L. Robinson, Anxiety responses to maximal exercise testing, *British Journal of Sports Medicine* 29 (1995): 97–102.

29. Similar results indicating increased anxiety for a short while following intense exercise followed by reduced anxiety was found by O'Connor et al., Anxiety responses.

30. Petruzzello, et al., A meta-analysis.

31. J. S. Raglin, P. E. Turner, and F. Eksten, State anxiety and blood pressure following 30 minutes of leg ergometry or weight training, *Medicine and Science in Sports and Exercise* 9 (1993): 1044–48.

32. P. J. O'Connor, C. X. Bryant, J. P. Veltri, and S. M. Gebhardt, State anxiety and ambulatory blood pressure following resistance exercise in females, *Medicine and Science in Sports and Exercise* 25 (1993): 516–21.

33. H. Selye, *The stress of life* (Toronto and London: McGraw-Hill, 1956).

34. D. C. McKenzie, Markers of excessive exercise, *Canadian Journal of Applied Physiology* 24 (1999): 66–73.

35. P. J. Beumont, B. Arthur, J. D. Russell, and S. W. Touyz, Excessive physical activity in eating disorder patients: Proposals for a supervised exercise program, *International Journal of Eating Disorders* 15 (1994): 21–36.

36. C. G. Long, J. Smith, M. Midgley, and T. Cassidy, Over-exercising in anorexic and normal samples: Behaviour and attitudes, *Journal of Mental Health* 2 (1993): 321–27.

37. E. McAuley, Physical activity and psychosocial outcomes, in *Physical activity, fitness, and health: international proceedings and consensus statement,* ed. C. Bouchard, R. J. Shephard and T. Stephens (Champaign, Ill.: Human Kenetics Publishers, 1994), and D. Scully, J. Kremer, M. M. Meade, R. Graham, and K. Dudgeon, Physical exercise and psychological well-being: A critical review, *British Journal of Sports Medicine* 32 (1998): 111–20.

38. In this research, twenty-three male and female college students completed measures of momentary self-esteem and AD ACL's (to assess energy and tension) multiple times over a seven-week period. A significant positive relationship was found between energy and self-esteem and a smaller, but still significant, negative correlation was found with tension (J. Rubadeau, The relationship between self-esteem, activation levels, and other situational determinants, Master's thesis, California State University, Long Beach, 1976).

39. McAuley, Physical activity and psychosocial outcomes; Scully, et al., Physical exercise and psychological well-being.

40. A. Bandura, Self-efficacy: Toward a unifying theory of behavior change, *Psychological Review* 84 (1977): 191–215.

41. McAuley, Physical activity and psychsocial outcomes; Scully, et al., Physical exercise and psychological well-being.

42. See Gauvin and Spence, Physical activity and psychological well-being, and Scully, et al., Physical exercise and psychological well-being.

43. See H. Osmond, R. Mullaly, and C. Bisbee, Mood pain: A comparative study of clinical pain and depression, *Journal of Orthomolecular Psychiatry* 14 (1985): 5–12.

44. See D. J. Crews and D. M. Landers, A meta-analytic review of aerobic fitness and reactivity to psychosocial stressors, *Medicine and Science in Sports and Exercise* 19 (1987): S114–20, and Scully, et al., Physical exercise and psychological well being.

45. A. Steptoe, J. Kimbell, and P. Basford, Exercise and the experience and appraisal of daily stressors: A naturalistic study, *Journal of Behavioral Medicine* 21 (1998): 363–74.

46. E. T. Hsiao and R. E. Thayer, Exercising for mood regulation: The importance of experience, *Personality and Individual Differences* 24 (1998): 829–36.

47. Richard Ryan and his associates at the University of Rochester clearly show that adherence to exercise is more likely to occur when physical activity has an intrinsic motivation. If it is intrinsically pleasurable, exercise will be continued, but extrinsic motivation—such as improved fitness or appearance—is associated with less adherence. See, for example, R. M. Ryan, C. M. Frederick, D. Lepes, N. Rubio, and K. M. Sheldon, Intrinsic motivation and exercise adherence, *International Journal of Sports Psychology* 28 (1997): 335–54.

48. In an interesting study showing that shorter periods of exercise often can be most effective, J. M. Jakicic and colleagues showed that individuals exercising in multiple short bouts per day, as compared to one continuous bout, had greater exercise adherence as well as a trend toward greater weight loss. Motivation to exercise probably underlies these findings (J. M. Jakicic, R. R. Wing, B. A. Butler, and R. J. Robertson, Prescribing exercise in multiple short bouts versus one continuous bout: Effects on adherence, cardiovascular fitness, and weight loss in overweight women, *International Journal of Obesity* 19 [1995]: 893–901).

49. J. M. Rippe and S. Hess, The role of physical activity in the prevention and management of obesity, *Journal of the American Dietetic Association* 98 (1998): S31–38.

50. In a review article, N. P. Pronk and R. R. Wing cite numerous studies that show that exercise is the single strongest predictor of weight loss maintenance across many types of people (Physical activity and long-term maintenance of weight loss, *Obesity Research* 2 [1994]: 587–99).

51. According to *McDonald's Nutrition Facts*, a Big Mac, large french fries, and medium Coke add up to 1,220 calories.

52. In a review, M. J. Toth and E. T. Poehlman concluded that exercise may be beneficial because of its preservative effect on daily energy expenditure, but that the paucity of studies prevents firm conclusions (Effects of exercise on daily energy expenditure, *Nutrition Reviews* 54 [1996]: S140–48). In another review of published evidence G. W. Gleim concluded that the role of exercise in maintaining resting metabolic rate for dieting women has only marginal support (Exercise is not an effective weight loss modality in women, *Journal of the American College of Nutrition* 12 [1993]: 363–67).

Chapter 4   Emotional Eating

1. Quotes are from jacket copy from the following books: R. Arnot, *Dr. Bob Arnot's revolutionary weight control program* (Boston: Little, Brown, 1997); R. Haas, *Eat smart, think smart* (New York: HarperCollins, 1994); E. Somer, *Food and mood* (New York: Holt, 1995); B. Sears, *The zone: A dietary road map* (New York: HarperCollins, 1995).

2. A random-digit telephone survey conducted in 1996 by state health departments showed that 28.8 percent of men and 43.6 percent of women were attempting to lose weight (M. K. Serdula, et al., Prevalence of attempting weight loss and strategies for controlling weight, *Journal of the American Medical Association* 282 [1999]: 1353–58).

3. It is a good idea to look at the Notes sections at the back of these books to see what kinds of citations of scientific studies are actually provided and not just claimed. See whether the studies support the central points that the author makes, or, as is often the case, whether they are just general references that sound authoritative and help make the book *appear* to be scientific. (Nowadays, with the availability of MedLine and PsycLIT in libraries and on the Internet, as well as other databases, it is usually possible at least to read the abstracts of cited scientific articles.) Too often we are told that "scientific studies show," or some such claim is made, but many times there are no citations of relevant studies. To convince the sophisticated reader, respected scientific journals should be cited, not just magazine articles or technical reports. Whenever possible, you should pay attention to bodies of scientific evidence, because a single study often doesn't hold up on replication. It isn't that there has been poor sci-

ence in that research, but each study has only a limited focus—a broader view may show something else.

4. It takes a while for good studies to be published, and sometimes there is a scientific snobbishness against some points of view that precludes studies even being done. I suggest that if you are a good self-observer and have a sense that a diet will work, you should try it and carefully watch your reactions for a couple of weeks. This isn't as good as a well-controlled scientific study, but some useful information may result, especially if you try to take into account your expectations and pay attention to other changes in your life that may occur at the same time as the diet, which may be the real causes for the different reactions you experience.

   In some respects these self-studies are even better than a large study done on average people because self-studies can take into account your uniqueness. (A type of research called *individual differences* focuses particularly on the ways that individuals vary, and this will be a subject later in the chapter.) What to pay attention to when observing the effects of a particular diet is crucial. Weight is important, but it must be lasting weight change. And mood is a key in management of appetite. See R. E. Thayer, *The biopsychology of mood and arousal* (New York: Oxford University Press, 1989), Chapter 7, for an extended discussion of methodology. For a discussion of other methodological issues, see L. B. Christensen, *Diet-behavior relationships* (Washington, D.C.: American Psychological Association, 1996).

5. There is something very seductive about food that is easily ingested as a solution to our problems. Any observer can note the huge attention to special-use foods in the commercial and media worlds. It is way out of proportion to simple nutrition needs. I suspect there is a deeper motivation for trying a special diet than comes only from the convenience of this practice. But this is perhaps understandable on a general biopsychological level, considering the necessity of food for life itself. Eating has an elemental significance, and that is likely to be reflected in our most basic tendencies and preferences.

6. D. Edell, with D. Schrieberg, *Eat, drink, and be merry* (New York: HarperCollins, 1999).

7. D. L. Watson and R. G. Tharp, *Self-directed behavior* (Pacific Grove, Calif.: Brooks/Cole, 1997).

8. The argument is not settled, however, even about how the intake of dietary fat—an energy-dense food—contributes to trends of increasing obesity. For example, in a recent exchange in the *American Journal of Clinical Nutrition*, W. C. Willett cited American eating trends toward reduced fat and various other ecological studies to question the conventional point of view that dietary fat is a major determinant of increasing obesity. In rebuttal, G. A. Bray and B. M. Popkin review a good deal of animal and clinical research, controlled trials, as well as ecological and epidemiological data to show that increased dietary fat produces obesity by increasing energy intake. See W. C. Willett, Dietary fat and obesity: An unconvincing relation, *American Journal of Clinical Nutrition* 68 (1998a): 1149–50; Is dietary fat a major determinant of body fat? *American Journal of Clinical Nutrition* 67 (1998b): 556S-62S; and G. A Bray and B. M. Popkin, Dietary fat does affect obesity! *American Journal of Clinical Nutrition* 68 (1998): 1157–73.

9. The usual figures of poor success at maintaining weight loss are controversial for various reasons, including the fact that they come from early studies and more important that failure rates are often computed from hard-core overweight people who take part in weight-loss programs and do not include those who have successfully managed weight loss on their own. Nonetheless, even optimistic success rates are disappointing. A good recent review of the issues and relevant studies is provided by W. C. Miller and A. K. Lindeman, The role of diet and exercise in weight management, in *Overweight and weight management,* ed. S. Dalton (Gaithersburg, Md.: Aspen Publishers, 1997).

10. R. M. Ganley, Emotion and eating in obesity: A review of the literature, *International Journal of Eating Disorders* 8 (1989): 342–61. Also see E. Abramson, *Emotional eating* (New York: Lexington Books, 1993), and a summary of a number of scales designed to measure emotional eating as well as a general discussion of the concept in M. S. Faith, D. B. Allison, and A. Geliebter, Emotional eating and obesity: Theoretical considerations and practical recommendations, in *Overweight and weight management,* ed. S. Dalton (Gaithersburg, Md.: Aspen Publishers, 1997).

11. The evidence is not without challenge, however. See for example, D. B. Allison and S. Heshka, Emotion and eating in obesity? A critical

analysis, *International Journal of Eating Disorders* 13 (1993): 289–95, and see a rebuttal of these ideas in T. Van Strien, In defense of psychosomatic theory: A critical analysis of Allison and Heshka's critical analysis, *International Journal of Eating Disorders* 17 (1995): 299–304. In some reviews, studies are listed in which emotional eating was not found, usually together with those where it was found. In those studies with no findings, emotional eating wasn't proved untrue; it simply wasn't observed. But it is well known among researchers in the field that it is easy to obtain no positive findings in a study. Poor methodology almost guarantees this outcome. Given the substantial amount of evidence that at least suggests emotional eating, I wonder whether the absence of a stronger acceptance of this concept could be influenced by its historical roots. Emotional eating is often traced to the so-called Psychosomatic Theory in historical analyses (H. Bruch, *Eating disorders: Obesity, anorexia nervosa, and the person within* [New York: Basic Books, 1973). This theory has a psychoanalytic history, and there is a distinct bias against psychoanalysis in modern-day scientific psychology. However, most current research on emotional eating, including most of that described in this book, has few or no direct psychoanalytic ties.

12. For hundreds of years, if not more, emotional eating was assumed (Bruch, *Eating disorders*), but demonstrating it is not easy. The best we usually can do is to ask people to keep track of their overeating and the moods they experience just before a binge or just before a diet is broken. Some studies just ask people to remember and describe those occasions, but more complex studies have sampled behavior on many occasions, for example, by getting reports from continuous diaries that experimental participants keep, or even by using a beeper to elicit systematic reports of emotional states just before eating. Some experiments manipulate or influence emotions without the experimental subject being aware of what is happening, and then "conveniently" provide snacks that can be eaten while researchers secretly observe how much is eaten. Generally we find that overeating and breaking diets are activities in which negative moods come first, but this isn't always found. As suggested, I believe that part of the reason many studies haven't shown this correlation is due to a methodological problem: emotions are hard to measure and even harder to change

in an experiment; exactly the right procedures must be used or there will be no findings. Due to these methodological shortcomings, it sometimes appears that there is no relationship between moods and overeating, although a relationship might be found if studied in a different way. This is one of the main arguments for the importance of self-study.

13. Issues of cause and effect are complex and are not dealt with definitively in this book. As will be seen in various studies to be described, negative moods reliably appear before overeating occurs and abate when the eating is under way or finished. Does this indicate that the negative moods have *caused* the overeating? Technically speaking, it probably would be best to refer to bodily processes that can be observed through our moods and the *apparent* influence on eating that these processes have. In subsequent chapters on mood, I will deal more with two kinds of general bodily arousal and the feelings or moods that are part of these arousal systems. These kinds of biopsychological arousal may be better understood in the causal sequence, but for now, my references to cause and effect are used in a more loose form.

14. A. J. Hill and L. Heaton-Brown, The experience of food craving: A prospective investigation in healthy women, *Journal of Psychosomatic Research* 38 (1994): 801–14.

15. H. P. Weingarten and D. Elston, Food cravings in a college population, *Appetite* 17 (1991): 167–75.

16. R. F. Baumeister, T. F. Heatherton, and D. M. Tice, *Losing control: How and why people fail at self-regulation* (San Diego, Calif.: Academic Press, 1994).

17. Chocolate also was the most craved food in the Weingarten and Elston study (Food cravings in a college population), especially among women.

18. In the mood checklist that was used (the UWIST), high hedonic tone is midway between high energetic arousal and low tense arousal, thus having characteristics of both.

19. Other empirical studies of the subjective accompaniments of hunger also show close associations with low energy and tension. For example, R. D. Mattes and M. I. Friedman, Hunger, *Digestive Diseases* 11 (1993): 65–77 used open-ended questionnaires to study hunger and

other subjective sensations among eighty-three males and females, and, after gastric growls and aches, a common accompaniment to hunger was "weakness" (low energy). "Anxiety" (tension) also was reported. J. Mayer, L. F. Monello, and C. C. Seltzer, Hunger and satiety sensation in man, *Postgraduate Medicine* 6 (1965): 97–102 tested 800 persons with a structured questionnaire and found that 80 percent of adults experienced weakness, tiredness, and restlessness, among other sensations, with extreme hunger, and, as deprivation increased, there was increasing frequency of what they called the triad of irritability, nervousness, and tenseness. In other words, these studies and others show that when you are hungry, some variation of tense tiredness usually is present. The primary origins of hunger are likely to be found in the brain, gut, liver, adipose tissue, and endocrine hormones (J. R. Vasselli and C. A. Maggio, Mechanisms of appetite and body weight regulation, in *Overweight and weight management,* ed. S. Dalton [Gaithersburg, Md.: Aspen Publishers, 1997]), but moods related to low energy and tension appear to be among the most prominent subjective signals that are aroused by deficits arising within the primary physiological systems. Motivation to eat is difficult to assess, but I believe that moods have an important motivating function. For example, as I have indicated, avoidance of unpleasant moods often motivates people to self-regulate with food.

20. Eating habits are established through reinforcement (for example, feeling better after ingestion of food), but there is a surprising absence of acknowledgment of this process in the eating research literature. I suspect it is because of the well-known phenomenon that people feel guilty after overeating, thus eating sugar and fat-filled foods appears to result in punishment rather than positive reinforcement—therefore, how could bad eating habits be learned? What is not recognized here, in my view, is that the positive feelings from eating occur almost immediately, whereas the guilt occurs a few seconds or minutes later. This may seem insignificant to those unfamiliar with the learning literature, but learning researchers have known for a long time that the immediacy of the reinforcer is very important in controlling the habit. The guilt is likely to have less effect on the eating habit than the positive feeling that occurred immediately. A second response to the guilt/punishment issue comes from a recent

study of binges that showed that the guilt experienced after a binge is less aversive than the relief from negative emotions that the bingeing produces (J. Kenardy, B. Arnow, and W. S. Agras, The aversiveness of specific emotional states associated with binge-eating in obese subjects, *Australian and New Zealand Journal of Psychiatry* 30 [1996]: 839–44).

21. Because the energy effects from food ingestion are subtle, they are difficult to demonstrate experimentally without very reliable measures. Nevertheless, there is a variety of evidence that indicates such effects exist. For example, in one experiment (R. E. Thayer, Energy, tiredness, and tension effects of a sugar snack versus moderate exercise, *Journal of Personality and Social Psychology* 52 [1987a]: 119–25), ingestion of a candy bar reliably resulted in increased energy over 30 minutes, followed by decreasing energy at 60 minutes and 120 minutes. Also relevant is research relating blood glucose level, subjective energy and tension (D. Benton and D. Owens, Is raised blood glucose associated with the relief of tension? *Journal of Psychosomatic Research* 37 [1993]: 723–735; A. E. Gold, K. M. MacLeod, I. J. Deary, and B. M. Frier, Changes in mood during acute hypoglycemia in healthy subjects, *Journal of Personality and Social Psychology* 68 [1995]: 498–504; D. S. Owens, P. Y. Parker, and D. Benton, Blood glucose and subjective energy following cognitive demand, *Physiology and Behavior* 62 [1997]: 471–78). And considering longer-term nutrition, the relationship of food intake and subjective energy is evident from studies of chronic starvation showing that energy declines with nutritional deficits (A. Keys, J. Brozek, A. Henschel, O. Mickelsen, and H. L. Taylor, *The biology of human starvation* [Minneapolis: University of Minnesota Press, 1950]). Also there are indirect confirmations from experiments that vary energy content of food, such as one in which desire to eat was influenced by a previously ingested low-energy breakfast and fullness by a high-energy breakfast (A. Lluch, P. Hubert, N. A. King, and J. E. Blundell, Selective effects of acute exercise and breakfast interventions on mood and motivation to eat, *Physiology and Behavior* 68 [2000]: 515–20).

22. S. Popless-Vawter, C. Brandau, and J. Straub, Triggers of overeating and related intervention strategies for women who weight cycle, *Applied Nursing Research* 11 (1998): 69–76.

23. Overeating sometimes occurs in the presence of positive moods, but the cause of this is not clear. Is it self-regulation of the type that occurs with negative moods, and, if so, how does this work? I previously hypothesized (*The origin of everyday moods* [New York: Oxford University Press, 1996]) that when a person is in a positive mood, there can still be minor variations in feelings of energy and tension— subtle dips in energy can be sensed, for example. These can motivate the person to reinstate to the fullest extent the positive feelings that she is experiencing. Moreover, the positive feelings being experienced can be so powerful as to counteract inhibitions against eating forbidden foods. In other words, the pleasure temporarily counteracts and eliminates the tension that maintains the inhibitions.

24. Popless-Vawter, Brandau, and Straub, Triggers of overeating. The researchers summed up their results as follows: "Unpleasant feelings of being tired, bored, lonely, anxious, tense, stressed, angry, and depressed were the emotional themes that appeared to stimulate women to overeat but were observed to a lesser extent in normal weight women. All women reported relief from unpleasant feelings while they were overeating except for obese subjects who reported a slight increase in anxiety (25% to 30%); this rise actually may not reflect an increase in their original unpleasant feelings but perhaps a rise in feeling guilty about overeating. Obese women mainly overate when they were tired, bored and lonely at the end of their work days. Considering overall averages, all subjects experienced fewer unpleasant feelings afterwards than before overeating. Obese women, however, reported feeling increased anger and depression, perhaps because of self-anger and disappointment about overeating" (page 74).

25. T. Tuomisto, M. T. Tuomisto, M. Hetherington, and R. Lappalainen, Reasons for initiation and cessation of eating in obese men and women and the affective consequences of eating in everyday situations, *Appetite* 30 (1998): 211–22.

26. This research appears to show that tense tiredness causes eating, but such logic is difficult to prove. The best we can do is to show that a particular feeling occurs just before eating, and that after eating the mood has changed. That happened here, but did the tense tiredness cause the eating? It seems likely because of the close association, and it also makes sense. We have learned in the past that food can raise our

energy and calm us. Incidentally, this kind of learning is easy because of the elemental biological relationship—energy-intensive food is a direct way of reducing the unpleasant feelings associated with tense tiredness. Scientists who study learning have found that biologically meaningful relationships are learned more readily than others. In any event, this research and other studies of this kind strongly suggest a causal relationship between tense tiredness and eating.

27. C. M. Grilo, S. Shiffman, and R. R. Wing, Relapse crises and coping among dieters, *Journal of Consulting and Clinical Psychology* 57 (1989): 488–95.

28. This third pattern when relapses occurred that these researchers called low arousal is a good indication of the motivation to seek energy by eating. Generally low arousal is a time when resources are depleted. It is often a period of needed recuperation, and if we must be active in a low arousal state, it can be a period of increased tension as well (Thayer, *Biopsychology of mood and arousal*).

29. R. R. Wing, S. Shiffman, R. G. Drapkin, C. M. Grilo, and M. McDermott, Moderate versus restrictive diets: Implications for relapse, *Behavior therapy* 26 (1995): 5–24.

30. D. J. LaPorte, A fatiguing effect in obese patients during partial fasting: Increase in vulnerability to emotion-related events and anxiety, *International Journal of Eating Disorders* 9 (1990): 345–55.

31. Since these anxiety measures were taken only once a week, they may not have been good indications of specific relapse episodes, but the fact that significant correlations occurred in the second half of the study even with such gross measures clearly indicates how one could have caused the other.

32. Researchers have been ingenious in figuring ways of determining the causes of overeating. One of the methodological questions that inevitably plagues diary studies of overeating (for example, diaries kept of relapses) is that the eating episodes that result in diary entries may be unique in some way, and episodes without diary entries may be different. C. Johnson and R. Larson set out to correct this deficiency by using pagers to randomly alert bulimic and normal women to report what they were doing and feeling at various times of day. One interesting result was that the bulimic women generally felt more irritable, sad, lonely, weak, and passive than the normal sub-

jects. This was determined by averaging all the momentary reports of the two groups. Thus, those who were often enveloped by the need to overeat experienced more negative moods overall, just the result you would expect if negative moods cause overeating. Another interesting finding was that the bulimic women reported significantly more times when they were thinking about, preparing, or eating food, compared to the normal women. Again, this suggests the importance of thoughts to overeating.

And what about the eating episodes themselves? Inevitably some of the times when the women were paged corresponded to binge-and-purge episodes. The times that these occurred illustrate a point I made earlier about how low bodily resources predispose us to overeat, a kind of drive to replenish our energy. The results showed that the food binges most often occurred in the afternoon and evenings. These are periods when energy reaches one of its low points of the day for most people. During these episodes the bulimic women reported that they were significantly more irritable and weak, and that they felt more constrained.

These results illustrate the tense-tired cause of overeating as a means of self-regulating. Of course, the participants in this research were limited to the rating scales provided for describing their feelings, and these did not include adjectives directly assessing tension, energy, or tiredness, but irritability and constrained feelings clearly are tension-related. And weakness is another way of describing low energy. Once again, overeating and tense tiredness are closely linked (C. Johnson and R. Larson, Bulimia: An analysis of moods and behavior, *Psychosomatic Medicine* 44 [1982]: 341–351).

33. American Psychiatric Association, *Diagnostic and statistical manual of mental disorders* (4th ed.) (Washington, D.C.: American Psychiatric Association, 1994).

34. G. G. Greeno and R. R. Wing, Stress-induced eating, *Psychological Bulletin* 115 (1994): 444–64.

35. D. B. Herzog, K. M. Nussbaum, and A. K. Marmor, Comorbidity and outcome in eating disorders, *The Psychiatric Clinics of North America* 19 (1996): 843–59.

36. J. E. Mitchell and M. P. Mussell, Comorbidity and binge eating disorder, *Addictive Behaviors* 20 (1995): 725–32.

37. S. R. Maddi, D. M. Khoshaba, M. Persico, F. Bleecker, G. VanArsdall, Psychosocial correlates of psychopathology in a national sample of the morbidly obese, *Obesity Surgery* 7 (1997): 397–404.

38. Greeno and Wing, Stress-induced eating. See also J. C. Barefoot, B. L. Heitmann, M. J. Helms, R. B. Williams, R. S. Surwit, and I. C. Siegler, Symptoms of depression and changes in body weight from adolescence to mid-life, *International Journal of Obesity and Related Metabolic Disorders* 22 (1998): 688–94; M. J. Garvey and C. B. Schaffer, Are some symptoms of depression age dependent? *Journal of Affective Disorders* 32 (1994): 247–51; and A. J. Stunkard, M. H. Fernstrom, R. A. Price, E. Buss, E. Frank, and D. J. Kupfer, Weight change in depression: Influence of "disinhibition" is mediated by body mass and other variables, *Psychiatry Research* 38 (1991): 197–200.

39. Thayer, *Biopsychology of mood and arousal.* This kind of analysis of stress reactions focuses on the moment-to-moment changes that can occur, while more traditional analyses focus on such long-term variables as temperament, usual coping style, and the presence or absence of social networks and supports. The latter influences may increase or decrease the stressful effect of any given activity or circumstance over time (cf. A. Steptoe, et al., The effect of life stress on food choice, in *"The nation's diet": The social science of food choice,* ed. A. Murcott [London: Longman, 1998]). But the moment-to-moment understanding of stress and the accompanying tension that it produces is much more useful for thinking about food urges and appetites, in my view.

40. This study provides a particularly reliable indication of how stress influences eating, since it doesn't depend on artificial laboratory manipulations of stressors. These manipulations can be ineffectual due to ethical constraints that prevent putting participants through really stressful conditions. On the other hand, in the day-to-day lives of these teachers and nurses, stress was a common occurrence. Moreover, the researchers compared the two weeks of the eight in which the most stress was registered by the nurses and teachers with the two weeks when there was the least stress. This kind of averaging gives a much more reliable approximation than when stress is assessed on only one occasion, a common practice in many laboratory studies (A. Steptoe, Z. Lipsey, and J. Wardle, Stress, hassles and varia-

tions in alcohol consumption, food choice and physical exercise: A diary study, *British Journal of Health Psychology* 3 [1998]: 51–63).

41. R. W. Jeffery and S. A. French, Epidemic obesity in the United States: Are fast foods and television viewing contributing? *American Journal of Public Health* 88 (1998): 277–80.

42. Steptoe, et al., Effect of life stress.

43. For other naturalistic examples, see B. S. McCann, R. Warnick, and H. Knopp, Changes in plasma lipids and dietary intake accompanying shifts in perceived workload and stress, *Psychosomatic Medicine* 52 (1990): 97–108, and C. I. Michaud, J. P. Kahn, N. Musse, C. Burlet, and J. P. Nicolas, Relationships between critical life events and eating behavior in high-school students, *Stress Medicine* 6 (1990): 57–64.

These naturalistic examples of the way eating habits change when stress arises contrast somewhat with mixed findings in laboratory studies using artificially produced stress delivered in a short period of time together with covert observations of how subjects may sample food offered them during the experiment (Greeno and Wing, Stress-induced eating).

In addition to much research with humans, Greeno and Wing also provide an excellent summary of many different studies concerning stress and eating among animals. In this research a variety of animals were subjected to stress and given an opportunity to eat. Most were rats, but in published research other animals were studied, including hamsters, cats, and even mollusks, slugs, and fish. Part of the problem in this kind of research is that scientists may not be sure that the kind of stressful conditions the animals were subjected to are comparable to what people experience under stress. Nonetheless, stress has been produced by tail pinching, electric shock, overcrowding, as well as other presumed stressors. In Greeno and Wing's summary of these studies, eleven experiments showed increased eating during or after stress, two were inconsistent, and one study showed no effect. Although lots of qualifications must be considered in these experiments, the overall results provide support for the contention that stressful conditions cause eating to increase. Incidentally, one of the qualifications noted in some experiments was that the stress-induced eating occurred only with some animals among the same species. This is a kind of individual difference that isn't understood, but it is interesting because in the next chapter we will consider some individual differences among humans that appear to predict well who will eat under stress. (Note: I don't do this kind of research with animals, but in my experience with other scientists who do, they usually make every attempt to ease any potential suffering that may occur.)

My evaluation of these various kinds of research puts greatest confidence in studies of the day-to-day stressors that most of us experience. These studies do not represent a single instance of stress, but rather prolonged stress that eventually takes its toll. In contrast, laboratory studies are usually based on weak stressors and generally take place in a short period of time—not nearly what is necessary to produce the kind of stress that turns us to high calorie food.

44. See C. P. Herman and D. Mack, Restrained and unrestrained eating, *Journal of Personality* 43 (1975): 647–60; T. F. Heatherton, C. P. Herman, J. Polivy, G. A. King, and S. T. McGree, The (mis)measurement of restraint: An analysis of conceptual and psychometric issues, *Journal of Abnormal Psychology* 97 (1998): 19–28; and R. G. Laessle, R. J. Tuschl, B. C. Kotthaus, and K. M. Pirke, A comparison of the validity of three scales for the assessment of dietary restraint, *Journal of Abnormal Psychology* 98 (1989): 504–7.

45. T. Rutledge and W. Linden, To eat or not to eat: Affective and physiological mechanisms in the stress-eating relationship, *Journal of Behavioral Medicine* 21 (1998): 221–40.

46. Another interesting part of this experiment was that Rutledge and Linden assessed blood pressure and heart rate while the subjects completed the cognitive tasks, and then the researchers correlated the physiological measures with eating. There was a significant negative correlation, with those subjects who were most physiologically aroused eating the least. These results support the idea outlined in the next chapter of alternative ways of dealing with hunger urges, such as short, brisk walks. Walks also create this kind of general physiological arousal and, as we have seen, temporarily reduce hunger.

47. In a review of studies on stress and eating by Greeno and Wing, which I mentioned previously, the researchers described eight studies that showed restrained eaters ate more while unrestrained eaters did not when the two groups were under stress, and this was compared to

one study in which the restrained eaters ate less. Notwithstanding the one study, this is a more or less consistent set of findings.

48. The Rutledge and Linden experiment is a good indication of this. The only ones who ate significantly more were those women who indicated by their mood ratings that the cognitive tasks were stressful. Why some of the participants in this experiment and in other similar experiments didn't eat more may be understood because the kind of innocuous stressors that are used in such studies are stressful only for those people already predisposed to be tense because of the attractive food. The unrestrained eaters, the nondieters, may not experience the experimental stressors as stressful at all, and therefore they will not be motivated to eat as a kind of self-regulation. Extending this logic to everyday situations, we may imagine that restrained eaters are constantly on guard against attractive food, and thus their tension level is heightened for this reason. Thayer, *Biopsychology of mood and arousal*.

49. B. Arnow, J. Kenardy, and W. S. Agras, The emotional eating scale: The development of a measure to assess coping with negative affect by eating, *International Journal of Eating Disorders* 18 (1995): 79–90; L. Christensen, *Diet-behavior relationships* (app. A) (Washington, D.C.: American Psychological Association, 1996); C. P. Herman and D. Mack, Restrained and unrestrained eating, *Journal of Personality* 43 (1975): 647–60; Heatherton, et al. (Mis)measurement of restraint; A. Steptoe, T. S. Pollard, and J. Wardle, Development of a measure of the motives underlying the selection of food: The food choice questionnaire, *Appetite* 25 (1995): 267–84; A. J. Stunkard and S. Messick, A three-factor eating questionnaire to measure dietary restraint, disinhibition and hunger, *Journal of Psychosomatic Research* 29 (1985): 71–83; and T. van Strien, J. E. R. Frijters, G. P. A. Bergers, and P. B. Defares, The Dutch eating behavior questionnaire (DEBQ) for assessment of restrained, emotional, and external eating behavior, *International Journal of Eating Disorders* 5 (1986): 295–315.

50. Early cross-sectional studies appeared to indicate no correlation between obesity and psychopathology involving depression and anxiety, but careful analyses of this research—taking into account methodological shortcomings of the earlier studies, as well as later studies with modern measurement techniques and better predictors

of how the psychopathology will show up—suggest that a correlation does exist. Because of the conflicting findings, however, it must be said that there is no certainty at this time. An extensive analysis of the research and the issues involved is presented in M. A. Friedman and K. D. Brownell, Psychological correlates of obesity: Moving to the next research generation, *Psychological Bulletin* 117 (1995): 3–20. They are more concerned with the effects of obesity on psychopathology than vice versa, but correlational studies usually do not make this causal distinction. In other words, studies showing a correlation between obesity and psychopathology can mean that either has caused the other.

51. Heredity continues to be among the most common explanations for obesity (for example, Bray, et al., 1992). However, although a genetic predisposition to overweight is highly likely, the mechanism by which this predisposition influences people is not well understood, and mood easily could have an important role in this influence (G. A. Bray, B. York, and J. DeLany, A survey of the opinions of obesity experts on the causes and treatment of obesity, *American Journal of Clinical Nutrition* 55 [1992]:151S-54S).

Chapter 5   Mood Pleasure: Food versus Exercise

1. J. Mayer, N. B. Marshall, J. J. Vitale, J. H. Christensen, M. B. Mashayekhi, and E. F. Stare, Exercise, food intake and body weight in normal rats and genetically obese adult mice, *American Journal of Physiology* 177 (1954): 544–48.

2. J. Mayer, R. Purnima, P. M. Kamikhya, Relation between caloric intake, body weight, and physical work: Studies in an industrial male population in West Bengal, *American Journal of Clinical Nutrition* 4 (1956): 169–75.

3. See R. E. Thayer, *The biopsychology of mood and arousal* (New York: Oxford University Press, 1989), and *The origin of everyday moods* (New York: Oxford University Press, 1996).

4. One exception, of course, may be seen in people suffering from anorexia nervosa who maintain their thin state with excessive exercise.

5. R. Andres, Body weight and age, in *Eating disorders and obesity: A com-*

prehensive handbook, ed. K. D. Brownell and C. G. Fairburn, 65–70, (New York: Guilford, 1995).

6. R. E. Thayer, D. P. Peters, P. J. Takahashi, and A. M. Birkhead-Flight, Mood and behavior (smoking and sugar snacking) following moderate exercise: A partial test of self-regulation theory, *Personality and Individual Differences* 14 (1993): 97–104.

7. The Activation-Deactivation Adjective Check List (AD ACL) was developed many years ago and has been used in hundreds of published scientific studies from laboratories around the world (language-translated versions), particularly ones in which the biopychological bases of mood are of interest. Thayer, *Biopsychology of mood and arousal,* app. 1, contains the best brief description of the test that measures energy, tension, tiredness, and calmness. Also see my website: www.csulb. edu/~thayer.

8. About a fourth of the time that meant reading, studying, or paperwork; another fourth or so watched TV; a third fourth attended a college lecture or listened to the radio or music. The remainder engaged in other sedentary activities.

9. N. A. King, V. J. Burley, and J. E. Blundell, Exercise-induced suppression of appetite: Effects on food intake and implications for energy balance, *European Journal of Clinical Nutrition* 48 (1994): 715–24.

10. A listing and review of other studies can be found in King, Burley, and Blundell, Exercise-induced suppression of appetite, and Thayer, et al., Mood and behavior (smoking and sugar snacking).

11. J. R. Vasselli and C. A. Maggio, Mechanisms of appetite and body weight regulation, in *Overweight and weight management*, ed. S. Dalton (Gaithersburg, Md.: Aspen Publishers, 1997).

12. R. M. Julien, *A primer of drug action* (New York: Freeman, 1992).

13. Quoted in G. Buchalter, "I fought for everything I got," *Parade* magazine, May 9, 1999, p. 5.

14. Thayer, *Biopsychology of mood and arousal: Origin of everyday moods.*

15. S. M. Hall, R. McGee, C. Tunstall, J. Duffy, and N. Benowitz, Changes in food intake and activity after quitting smoking, *Journal of Consulting and Clinical Psychology* 57 (1989): 81–86.

16. National Task Force on the Prevention and Treatment of Obesity, Long-term pharmacotherapy in the management of obesity, *Journal of the American Medical Association* 276 (1996): 1907–15.

17. L. H. Brauer, C. E. Johanson, C. R. Schuster, R. B. Rothman, and H. de Wit, Evaluation of phentermine and fenfluramine, alone and in combination, in normal, healthy volunteers, *Neuropsychopharmacology* 14 (1996): 233–241.

18. As Dr. Judith Rodin points out in her excellent book *Body traps* (New York: Morrow, 1992), a marketing research firm calculated that Americans spent $33 billion on diets and diet-related services in 1990, and the trend is up.

19. See S. O. Cousins. *Exercise, aging, and health* (New York: Taylor and Francis, 1998).

20. Extensive surveys in the Surgeon General's report on physical activity and health show that, for those eighteen years of age and above reporting no participation in leisure time physical activity, percentages invariably increase with age. In addition, women report less leisure-time physical activity than do men, and less activity is reported by those with lower education and less income (*Physical activity and health: A report of the surgeon general*, Atlanta, Ga.: U.S. Department of Health and Human Services, Centers for Disease Control and Prevention, National Center for Chronic Disease Prevention and Health Prevention, President's Council on Physical Fitness and Sports, 1996).

21. T. Stephens and C. L. Craig, *The well-being of Canadians: Highlights of the 1988 Campbell's Survey* (Ottawa: Canadian Fitness and Lifestyle Research Institute, 1990).

22. As cited in Rodin, *Body traps,* p. 172.

Chapter 6   Why Do We Have Moods?

1. Serious depressions can last longer, of course. For example, the diagnostic criteria for Major Depressive Episode in *DSM-IV* involve five or more symptoms that have been present during the same two-week period and represent a change from previous functioning (at least one of the symptoms is either depressed mood or loss of interest or pleasure).

2. Although moods are usually associated with emotional states, the term can be use to refer to cognitive predispositions, as in, "I am in a serious or concentrative *mood*." Also, the word mood sometimes is

used to refer to a predisposition to do something, as in, "I am in the *mood* for some ice cream" (R. E. Thayer, *The biopsychology of mood and arousal* [New York: Oxford University Press, 1989]).

3. R. Ketai, Affect, mood, emotion and feeling: Semantic considerations, *American Journal of Psychiatry* 132 (1975): 1215–17; H. Owens and J. S. Maxmen, Mood and affect: A semantic confusion, *American Journal of Psychiatry* 136 (1979): 97–99.

4. In some of my early research, clear relationships were shown between verbal reports of moods and physiological measures of these states. See R. E. Thayer, Activation states as assessed by verbal report and four psychophysiological variables, *Psychophysiology* 7 (1970): 86–94.

5. D. M. McNair, M. Lorr, and L. F. Droppleman, *Manual: profile of mood states* (San Diego, Calif.: Educational and Industrial Testing Service, 1971).

6. The most complete description of the AD ACL, but without psychometric statistics, can be found in R. E. Thayer, *The biopsychology of mood and arousal* (New York: Oxford University Press, 1989), app. 1. Also see my website: www.csulb.edu/~thayer.

7. See V. Nowlis, Research with the Mood Adjective Check List, in *Affect, cognition, and personality*, ed. S. S. Tomkins and C. E. Izard, 352–89 (New York: Springer, 1965); V. Nowlis and H. H. Nowlis, The description and analysis of moods, *Annals of the New York Academy of Science* 65 (1956): 345–55.

8. J. A. Russell, A circumplex model of affect, *Journal of Personality and Social Psychology* 39 (1980): 1161–78; M. S. M. Yik, J. A. Russell, and L. F. Barrett, Structure of self-reported current affect: Integration and beyond, *Journal of Personality and Social Psychology* 77 (1999): 600–619.

9. D. Watson and A. Tellegen, Toward a consensual structure of mood, *Psychological Bulletin* 98 (1985): 219–35.

10. In their 1999 article, Watson, Tellegen, and their associates describe Positive Activation and Negative Activation as showing the close affinity to my dimensions of Energetic Arousal and Tense Arousal (D. Watson, D. Wiese, J. Vaidya, and A. Tellegen, Two general activation systems of affect: Structural findings, evolutionary considerations, and psychobiological evidence, *Journal of Personality and Social Psychology* 76 (1999): 820–38.

11. G. Matthews and his associates have adopted my concepts of Energetic and Tense Arousal, but in addition they posit a third dimension called Hedonic Tone, which is roughly comparable to Russell's pleasure dimension and my calm energy. R. J. Larsen and E. Diener have proposed dimensions similar to Russell's, but with certain variations. And D. P. Green, S. L. Goldman, and P. Salovey, have argued that the elimination of measurement errors together with multiple assessments changes the polar opposites of various dimensions proposed by others (G. Matthews, D. M. Jones, and A. G. Chamberlain, Refining the measurement of mood: The UWIST Mood Adjective Checklist, *British Journal of Psychology* 81 [1990]: 17–42; R. J. Larsen and E. Diener, Promises and problems with the circumplex model of emotion, in *Review of personality and social psychology: Emotion,* vol. 13, ed. M. S. Clark, 25–59 [Newbury Park, Calif.: Sage, 1992]; D. P. Green, S. L. Goldman, and P. Salovey, Measurement error masks bipolarity in affect ratings, *Journal of Personality and Social Psychology* 64 [1993]: 1029–41).

12. For example, see W. P. Morgan and M. L. Pollock, Psychological characterization of the elite distance runner, *Annals of the New York Academy of Science* 301 (1978): 382–403.

13. See, for example, S. Suzuki, *Zen mind, beginner's mind* (New York: Weatherhill, 1970).

14. See F. Farley, The big T in personality, *Psychology Today* 20 (1986): 44–52; M. Friedman and R. H. Rosenman, *Type A behavior and your heart* (New York: Knopf, 1974); R. A. Hicks, J. Green, and J. Haleblian, The Thayer Scale response patterns of Type A and Type B college students, *Psychological Reports* 65 (1989): 1167–70.

15. L. A. Clark and D. Watson, Tripartite model of anxiety and depression: Psychometric evidence and taxonomic implications, *Journal of Abnormal Psychology* 100 (1991): 316–36.

16. Larry Mantel's *Air Talk,* KPPC, Pasadena, Calif., July 3, 1996.

17. For example, see the January 2000 issue of *The American Psychologist,* which is devoted entirely to happiness, excellence, and optimal human functioning (Editors: Martin Seligman and Mihaly Csikszentmihalyi). See also two recent books for general audiences: S. Braun, *The science of happiness* (New York: Wiley, 2000), and D. Lykken, *Happiness: What studies of twins show us about nature, nurture and the happiness set-point* (New York: Golden Books, 1999).

18. See Yik, Russell, and Barrett, Structure of self-reported current affect.

19. This relationship between happiness and calm energy is consistent with the tendency of extraverts to be more energetic and the tendency of those high in neuroticism to be more tense (P. T. Costa and R. R. McCrae, Influence of extraversion and neuroticism on subjective well-being: Happy and unhappy people, *Journal of Personality and Social Psychology* 38 [1980]: 668–78; H. J. Eysenck and M. W. Eysenck, *Personality and individual differences: A natural science approach* [New York: Plenum, 1985]).

20. K. M. DeNeve and H. Cooper, The happy personality: A meta-analysis of 137 traits and subjective well-being, *Psychological Bulletin* 124 (1998): 197–229.

21. Michael Robinson provides persuasive evidence that the way life circumstances affect cognitive well-being is through their influence on mood. This supports my argument that mood states represent important signal systems that give us vital information about our momentary condition (M. D. Robinson, The reactive and prospective functions of mood: Its role in linking daily experiences and cognitive well-being, *Cognition and Emotion* 14 [2000]: 145–76).

22. E. Diener, H. Smith, and F. Fujita, The personality structure of affect, *Journal of Personality and Social Psychology* 69 (1995): 130–41.

23. C. Tavris, *Anger: The misunderstood emotion,* rev. ed. (New York: Simon & Schuster, 1989).

24. See R. M. Nesse, The evolution of hope and despair, *Social Research* 66 (1999): 429–69, for another, but somewhat similar, analysis of the functions of moods.

25. In *Biopsychology of mood and arousal,* p. 64, I discuss several possible adaptive functions for the conscious awareness of moods. These include multilevel nervous system organization, with an executive or planning function superseding lower levels. Or possibly the adaptive function involves human language and the ability to communicate information about moods to others.

26. One of my students and I studied the relationship between skilled mental performance and mood, with the help of nine students who occasionally stopped their reading and studying on many occasions over a three-week period and rated the effectiveness of their recent

mental work. At the same time they rated their moods (AD ACLs). Calm energy was the best predictor of study effectiveness; tense energy was the next best pattern; and tense tiredness was the worst. These differences were highly reliable (F. M. Docuyanan and R. E. Thayer, *Effectiveness of study time as a function of transitory moods,* paper presented at the annual convention of the American Psychological Association, Toronto, Canada, 1993).

27. A. Bandura, Self-efficacy: Toward a unifying theory of behavior change, *Psychological Review* 84 (1977): 191–215.
28. See Clark and Watson, Tripartite model of anxiety and depression.
29. As I have indicated, most scientists agree there are two (possibly three) major dimensions of mood, variously called Positive and Negative Affect, Pleasantness and Activation, and Energetic and Tense Arousal. One of the reasons I believe that the foundations of mood lie in energetic and tense arousal is the obvious biological underpinning for these two arousal systems. Other analyses are generally based on self-reports of mood—which can be valuable, as well as having great practical use, but biological underpinnings are more convincing when we search for the basic origins of mood. There is also another way in which energetic and tense arousal differ from other self-report theories about the dimensions of mood, and this has to do with the way that energy and tension seem to influence each other in a complex pattern. These formularized interactions are so fundamental, and they occur in such different social contexts, as to strongly suggest a biological basis.

   In technical terms, it appears that measures of tension and energy are positively correlated between low and moderate arousal levels. But as tension increases further, the two kinds of arousal become negatively correlated at some point. The same pattern of positive and negative correlations occurs with different levels of *energy.* That is, up to moderate levels, energy and tension are positively correlated, but from moderate to high levels of energy, the two are negatively correlated. In the text I speak of tension as first causing energy to increase and then, at high levels, reducing energy, but this kind of cause-and-effect relationship is yet to be proved in experimental studies. At best, we can demonstrate positive and negative correlations between tension and energy measures at different levels of arousal.

This complex relationship between energetic and tense arousal relates to other issues that currently are prominent in mood research as well. Many scientists argue that the two systems of mood that have been identified are essentially independent, but the proof of this independence exists only in *cross-sectional studies,* not in studies of mood change. That is, if you take a large group of people and measure their mood at one time, you find good moods, neutral moods, and bad moods, and when you compare all the moods at once using a mathematical technique for summary descriptions called factor analysis, good moods and bad moods *appear* to be independent of each other. (See challenges to the concept of independence, however, in D. P. Green and P. Salovey, In what sense are positive and negative affect independent? A reply to Tellegen, Watson, and Clark, *Psychological Science* 10 [1999]: 304–6, and elsewhere.) It is this kind of summary comparison that leads supporters of positive and negative affect to argue that the two mood systems are independent. Another argument in the scientific literature holds that if the two are independent, then you have the apparently untenable position that a person can experience both positive and negative affect (or activation) at the same time!

I believe that this appearance of independence is wrong when changing moods are considered. If they are measured cross-sectionally, energetic and tense arousal states appear to be independent, just as the other mood systems do, but because of the positive and negative correlations described here, this assumption of independence is wrong. Moods change constantly, and the best conceptualization of them shows that they influence each other at different levels of arousal.

30. See N. Kleitman, *Sleep and wakefulness (revised and enlarged edition)* (Chicago: University of Chicago Press, 1963), and E. J. Murray, *Sleep, dreams, and arousal* (New York: Appleton-Century-Crofts, 1965).

31. Thayer, *Biopsychology of mood and arousal.*

Chapter 7 Changes in Energy—and Mood

1. Feelings of energy can be understood in relation to the Activation-Deactivation Adjective Check List. See R. E. Thayer, *The origin of everyday moods* (New York: Oxford University Press, 1996), app. 1.

Also see my website: www.csulb.edu/~thayer. The Energy subtest includes the common elements of the following five adjectives: active, energetic, vigorous, lively, full of pep.

2. So-called ultradian rhythms of ninety minutes have been observed in a variety of functions, including sleepiness, EEG, daydreaming, vigilance, and even hypnotizability. REM cycles could be the most primitive indication of this 90–minute pattern (see references in R. E. Thayer, *The biopsychology of mood and arousal* [New York: Oxford University Press, 1989]).

3. These patterns have been observed. See R. E. Thayer, Toward a psychological theory of multidimensional activation (arousal), *Motivation and Emotion* 2 (1978b): 1–34; R. E. Thayer, Problem perception, optimism, and related states as a function of time of day (diurnal rhythm) and moderate exercise: Two arousal systems in interaction, *Motivation and Emotion* 11 (1987b): 19–36; R. E. Thayer, P. J. Takahashi, and J. A. Pauli, Multidimensional arousal states, diurnal rhythms, cognitive and social processes, and extraversion, *Personality and Individual Differences* 9 (1988): 15–24.

4. As an example of recent research on this kind of cycle, C. Czeisler and associates at Harvard Medical School argue that the intrinsic period of the human circadian pacemaker is 24.18 hours, rather than the slightly longer period previously assumed. This cycle presumably is controlled by the suprachiasmatic nucleus of the brain (C. A. Czeisler, et al., Stability, precision, and near-24–hour period of the human circadian pacemaker, *Science* 284 (1999): 2177–81).

5. Additionally, as I mentioned earlier, various *ultradian cycles* (less than twenty-four hours) have been associated with mood. I reviewed and referenced much of that scientific literature in my earlier two books, *The biopsychology of mood and arousal* and *The origin of everyday moods* (New York: Oxford University Press, 1989, 1996).

6. A pattern of higher depression (and increased tension) upon awakening has been documented in some clinical cases, and in the past this morning depression was one of the classic diagnostic indications of what was then called melancholia. As with other psychiatric observations, however, different patterns have been observed, and the current DSM-IV psychiatric classification system does not employ the morning pattern as a symptom of major depression.

7. For the first report on this syndrome, see A. J. Stunkard, W. J. Grace, and H. G. Wolff, The night-eating syndrome: A pattern of food intake among certain obese patients, *American Journal of Medicine* 19 (1955): 78–86. For a current review, see N. J. Aronoff, Obesity-related eating patterns: Binge-eating disorder and the night-eating syndrome, in *Overweight and weight management,* ed. S. Dalton (Gaithersburg, Md.: Aspen Publishers, 1997).

8. See C. S. W. Rand, A. M. C. Macgregor, and A. J. Stunkard, The night eating syndrome in the general population and among postoperative obesity surgery patients, *International Journal of Eating Disorders* 22 (1997): 65–69, and A. J. Stunkard, Binge-eating disorder and the night-eating syndrome, *International Journal of Obesity* 20 (1996): 1–6.

9. Aronoff, Obesity-related eating patterns.

10. See Thayer, *Biopsychology of mood and arousal* and *Origin of everyday moods,* and also P. H. Blaney, Affect and memory: A review, *Psychological Bulletin* 99 (1986): 229–46.

11. Thayer, Problem perception.

12. Compare L. Gauvin, W. J. Rejeski, and B. A. Reboussin, Contributions of acute bouts of vigorous physical activity to explaining diurnal variations in feeling states in active, middle-aged women, *Health Psychology* 19 (2000): 365–75.

13. For a variety of research approaches to cognition and mood, see D. M. Wegner and J. W. Pennebaker, eds., *Handbook of mental control* (Englewood Cliffs, N.J.: Prentice-Hall, 1993). For the cognitive theory of depression, A. T. Beck, *Cognitive therapy and the emotional disorders* (New York: International Universities Press, 1976).

14. R. E. Thayer, J. R. Newman, and T. M. McClain, The self-regulation of mood: Strategies for changing a bad mood, raising energy, and reducing tension, *Journal of Personality and Social Psychology* 67 (1994): 910–25.

15. See S. K. Nolen-Hoeksema, *Women and depression* (Stanford, Calif.: Stanford University Press, 1990), as well as a good deal of later research by this scientist.

16. Thayer, *Origin of everyday moods.*

17. When we study the mood of people who momentarily feel sociable, we find that this feeling is closely correlated with feeling energetic (W. Revelle, Manipulations and measurement of arousal: Within and

between—Subject evidence for two components of arousal, paper presented at the meeting of the International Society for the Study of Individual Differences, Baltimore, Md., 1993). I am not saying that they are the same, but careful psychometric studies show that when people feel sociable, they also feel energetic.

18. For example, A. Smith and his colleagues in the United Kingdom recently provided objective evidence that having a cold is associated with reduced alertness (alertness is correlated energy) and slowed reaction time (A. Smith, M. Thomas, J. Kent, and K. Nicholson, Effects of the common cold on mood and performance, *Psychoneu-roendocrinology* 23 [1998]: 733–39).

19. D. Buchwald, J. L. Sullivan, and A. L Komaroff, Frequency of 'chronic active Epstein-Barr virus infection' in general medical practice, *Journal of the American Medical Association* 257 (1987): 2303–7.

20. J. K. Dixon, J. P. Dixon, and M. Hickey, Energy as a central factor in the self-assessment of health, *Advances in Nursing Science* 15 (1993): 1–12.

21. S. Cohen, D. A. J. Tyrrell, and A. P. Smith, Psychological stress and susceptibility to the common cold, *New England Journal of Medicine* 325 (1991): 606–12.

22. S. Cathcart and D. Pritchard, Relationship between arousal-related moods and episodic tension-type headache: A biopsychological study, *Headache* 38 (1998): 214–21.

23. S. Maier and L. Watkins present persuasive evidence for the interesting theory that the immune system is a kind of bodily sense organ that even predates the fight-or-flight response in evolutionary history. This defense against infection activates the brain in basic ways (see Chapter 8). They even suggest that some forms of depression may be linked to immune system response (S. F. Maier and L. R. Watkins, The immune system as a sensory system: Implications for psychology, *Current Directions in Psychological Science* 9 [2000]: 98–102).

24. See A. A. Stone, et al., Evidence that secretory IgA antibody is associated with daily mood, *Journal of Personality and Social Psychology* 52 (1987): 988–93. See also A. A. Stone, J. M. Neale, D. S. Cox, A. Napoli, H. Valdimarsdottir, and E. Kennedy-Moore, Daily events are associated with secretory immune response to an oral antigen in men, *Health Psychology* 13 (1994): 440–46.

25. H. B. Valdimarsdottir and D. H. Bovbjerg, Positive and negative mood: Association with natural killer cell activity, *Psychology and Health* 12 (1997): 319–27.

26. For the negative effects of modest sleep loss see M. Irwin, et al., Partial night sleep deprivation reduces natural killer and cellular immune responses in humans, *Journal of the Federation of the American Societies for Experimental Biology* 10 (1996): 643–53. The relationship between sleep loss and immune system functioning is not without conflicting findings however, as is evident in D. F. Dingus, S. D. Douglas, S. Hamarman, L. Zaugg, and S. Kapoor, Sleep deprivation and human immune function, *Advances in Neuroimmunology* 5 (1995): 97–110.

27. W. C. Dement, *The promise of sleep* (New York: Delacorte Press, 1999); J. B. Maas, *Power sleep* (New York: Villard, 1998).

28. Dement, *The promise of sleep*, p. 276.

29. D. F. Dingus, et al., Cumulative sleepiness, mood disturbance, and psychomotor vigilance performance decrements during a week of sleep restricted to 4–5 hours per night, *Sleep* 20 (1997): 267–77.

30. This is evident from a statistical (meta)analysis of the results of nineteen original studies by J. Pilcher and A. Hoffcutt, sleep scientists from Bradley University (J. J. Pilcher, A. I. Huffcutt, Effects of sleep deprivation on performance: A meta-analysis, *Sleep* 19 [1996]: 318–26).

31. *Wake up America: A national sleep alert,* vol. 1 of Report of the National Commission on Sleep Disorders Research (Washington, D.C.: U.S. Department of Health and Human Services, 1993).

32. Gallup poll (ending date: July 21, 1996); Princeton Survey Research poll (ending date: November 15, 1994); Harris poll (ending date: December 13, 1989); Harris poll (ending date: March 15, 1984); Gallup poll (ending date: April 12, 1947).

33. Spaniards are gradually succumbing to modern-day time demands, unfortunately, and siestas are on the decline. Regular siesta-takers were reduced by 24 percent in one nationwide survey (*Los Angeles Times*, March 28, 2000).

34. In considering the topic of sleep and mood, I should mention one matter about sleep deprivation that sometimes is prominent in the news. A number of studies have now demonstrated that one night of sleep deprivation, or several nights of substantial but not complete

deprivation, can lead to a temporary remission of depression. As with other factors affecting mood, individual differences must be taken into account—in this case, whether the person is seriously depressed. Also, while a night or two of partial sleep deprivation—say, getting up at 1:00 A.M.—may be effective in relieving serious depression, no one knows why. It could be a shock to the system that disrupts physiological patterns that have developed and that maintain the depression, and in that respect it might be similar to the positive effects of electroconvulsive shock that are sometimes observed to relieve episodes of serious depression. Nevertheless, chronic sleep deprivation such as many people experience is much more likely to have an overall negative effect on mood and on low-level depression. For more on beneficial effects of sleep deprivation, see T. A. Wehr, Effects of wakefulness and sleep on depression and mania, in *Sleep and biological rhythms,* ed. J. Montplaisir and R. Godbout (New York: Oxford University Press, 1990), 42–86.

Also note the recent research on the effect of sleep deprivation on depressed people using PET (positive electron tomography) scans, a procedure that shows activity in different parts of the brain. Those patients with significant response to the deprivation had higher metabolic rates in the medial prefrontal cortex (see Chapter 8 herein), ventral anterior cingulate, and posterior subcallosal gyrus (J. Wu, et al., Prediction of antidepressant effects of sleep deprivation by metabolic rates in the ventral anterior cingulate and medial prefrontal cortex, *American Journal of Psychiatry* 156 [1999]: 1149–58).

35. Although there is usually a cognitive intermediary between a stimulus and our tense reaction, there are times when tense arousal appears to occur more directly. Consider, for example, pain generated in a dentist's office that results in muscle tension as you react. Or you may wake up with tense muscles from some physical disturbance that occurred during sleep. For further discussion of this matter, see Thayer, *Biopsychology of mood and arousal.*

36. R. J. Lazarus, *Emotion and adaptation* (New York: Oxford University Press, 1991).

37. R. A. Wright and J. W. Brehm, Energization and goal attractiveness, in *Goal concepts in personality and social psychology,* ed. L. A. Pervin (Hillsdale, N.J.: Erlbaum, 1989), 169–210.

Chapter 8   The Biopsychology of Energy and Tension

1. Walter Cannon, the scientist who developed the concept of the fight-or-flight response, recognized that fear may be paralyzing until there is "definite deed to perform" (W. B. Cannon, *Bodily changes in pain, hunger, fear and rage* [New York: Harper & Row, 1929/1963], p. 198).

2. Note, for example, K. M. Dillon, Popping sealed-air capsules to reduce stress, *Psychological Reports* 71(1992): 243–46.

3. See T George Harris's prescription for relaxation that combines the energizing effect of walking with the tension-reducing effect of a prayer mantra: L. Mundy, contributing ed. T George Harris, *The complete guide to prayer-walking: A simple path to body-and-soul fitness* (St. Meinrad, Ind.: Abbey Press, 1994).

4. See C. S. Carver, S. K. Sutton, and M. F. Scheier, Action, emotion and personality: Emerging conceptual integration, *Personality and Social Psychology Bulletin* 26 (2000): 741–51.

5. For example, J. L. Hager used stress films versus a brief period of vigorous exercise to study respiration patterns. There was arousal in both groups, but exercisers breathed more deeply, while those who were stressed breathed fast and shallowly (J. L. Hager, The human respiratory response in state anxiety, Ph.D. diss., Cornell University, *Dissertation Abstracts International* 37 [1976]: 5423B).

6. For a recent review, see T. M. Field, Massage therapy effects, *American Psychologist* 53 (1998): 1270–81.

7. Muscle relaxation in various forms is a time-honored technique that is widely used in stress management, and thus to relieve tension. Years ago the physician Edmond Jacobson extensively studied this form of relaxation and published his observations and advice in a series of popular books, most notably *Anxiety and tension control* (Philadelphia: Lippincott, 1964). Jacobson's books were read and used effectively by large numbers of people, and although now they may be out of print, they continue to be a valuable resource. His methods often are cited in the behavioral and stress-management literature. In more recent books, whenever tension reduction is under consideration, such methods as active or passive muscle relaxation and progressive muscle relaxation are central techniques (for example, D. L. Watson and R. G. Tharp, *Self-directed behavior* [Pacific Grove, Calif.: Brooks/Cole, 1997]).

8. D. Benton and D. Owens, Is raised blood glucose associated with the relief of tension? *Journal of Psychosomatic Research* 37 (1993): 723–35.

9. A. C. Gold, K. M. Macleod, I. Deary, and B. M. Frier, Changes in mood during acute hypoglycemia in healthy subjects, *Journal of Personality and Social Psychology* 68 (1995): 498–504; D. A. Hepburn, I. J. Deary, M. Munoz, and B. M. Frier, Physiological manipulations of psychometric mood factors using acute insulin-induced hypoglycemia in humans, *Personality and Individual Differences* 18 (1995): 385–91.

10. Recently this research group (McCrimmon, Frier, and Deary) used insulin manipulation to show effects on cognition from tense-tiredness, a relationship discussed in Chapter 7 herein (R. J. McCrimmon, B. M. Frier, and I. J. Deary, Appraisal of mood and personality during hypoglycaemia in human subjects, *Physiology and Behavior* 67 [1999]: 27–33).

11. J. A. Hobson, *The chemistry of conscious states* (Boston: Little, Brown, 1994), p. 184.

12. Personal communication, September 2, 1994.

13. R. A. Dienstbier, Arousal and physiological toughness: Implications for mental and physical health, *Psychological Review* 96 (1989): 84–100.

14. W. D. McArdle, F. I. Katch, and V. L. Katch, *Exercise physiology: Energy nutrition and human performance* (Philadelphia: Lea and Febiger, 1991).

15. R. A. Dienstbier, Behavioral correlates of sympathoadrenal reactivity: The toughness model, *Medicine and Science in Sports and Exercise* 23 (1991): 846–52.

16. For example, see M. M. van Eck and N. A. Nicolson, Perceived stress and salivary cortisol in daily life, *Annals of Behavioral Medicine* 16 (1994): 221–27.

17. P. Peeke, *Fight fat after forty* (New York: Viking, 2000).

18. T. W. Castonguay, Glucocorticoids as modulators in the control of feeding. *Brain Research Bulletin* 27 (1991): 423–28.

19. E. R. Kandel, Disorders of mood: Depression, mania, and anxiety disorders, in *Principles of neural science*, ed. E. R. Kandel, et al., 869–86 (Norwalk, Conn.: Appleton and Lange, 1991).

20. G. M. Pepper and D. T. Krieger, Hypothalamic-pituitary-adrenal

abnormalities in depression: Their possible relation to central mechanisms regulating ACTH release, in *Neurobiology of Mood Disorders,* ed. R. M. Post and J. C. Ballenger (Baltimore: Williams and Wilkens, 1984). One physiological test that has been used to diagnose depression is the dexamethasone suppression test (DST). About half the patients with major depressive disorders show a lack of cortisol suppression by normal inhibitory processes in the body following an earlier injection of the synthetic steroid dexamethasone (W. A. Brown, Use of dexamethasone suppression test in test of depression, in *Neurobiology of mood disorders,* ed. P. M. Post and J. C. Ballenger [Baltimore: Williams and Wilkens, 1984]). This indicates that the body does not adequately control cortisol levels. On the other hand, nondepressed persons show normal suppression. There has been some hope that the DST would be the long-sought physiological test of depression; unfortunately, it has not proved to be a conclusive indicator because many people diagnosed with depression have a negative DST result.

21. See, for example, J. E. Zweifel and W. H. O'Brien, A meta-analysis of the effect of hormone replacement therapy upon depressed mood, *Psychoneuroendocrinology* 22 (1997): 189–212.

22. I. M. Jackson, The thyroid axis and depression, *Thyroid* 8 (1998): 951–56.

23. R. L. Hoffman, *Intelligent medicine* (New York: Simon & Schuster, 1997).

24. C. B. Pert, *Molecules of emotion* (New York: Scribner, 1997), p. 25.

25. Ibid.

26. A little help from serotonin, *Newsweek,* January 5, 1998.

27. B. L. Jacobs and E. C. Azmitia, Structure and function of the brain serotonin system, *Physiological Reviews* 72 (1992): 165–229. The central brain stem raphe cell system, where serotonin originates, is the most expansive and complex neurochemical system in the CNS of mammals. Serotonin fibers project upwardly to the cerebral cortex and down to the tip of the spinal cord. Although they comprise only a few hundred thousand neurons among the millions of neurons of the nervous system, their influence is inordinately great. Each neuron exerts an influence over as many as 500,000 target neurons. For a readable and authoritative description of serotonin, see B. L. Jacobs,

Serotonin, motor activity and depression-related disorders, *American Scientist* 82 (1994): 456–63.

28. See, for example, B. E. Leonard, Serotonin receptors and their function in sleep, anxiety disorders and depression, *Psychotherapy and Psychosomatics* 65 (1996): 66–75.

29. P. Stark and C. D. Hardison, A review of multicenter controlled studies of Fluoxetine vs. Imipramine and placebo in outpatients with Major Depressive Disorder, *Journal of Clinical Psychiatry* 46 (1985): 53–58. See also P. E. Stokes, Fluoxetine: A five-year review, *Clinical Therapeutics* 15 (1993): 216–43.

30. D. O. Antonuccio, W. G. Danton, and G. Y. DeNelsky, Psychotherapy versus medication for depression: Challenging the conventional wisdom with data, *Professional Psychology: Research and Practice* 26 (1995): 574–85; I. Kirsch and G. Sapirstein, Listening to Prozac but hearing placebo: A meta-analysis of antidepressant medication, *Prevention and Treatment* 1 (1998). While it is apparent that antidepressants do help, they are not as effective as strong advocates sometimes seem to suggest. In a recent online survey of patients who were then taking antidepressants or had taken them in the past five years, conducted by the National Depressive and Manic-Depressive Association, 81 percent indicated that their depression continued to impair their social lives moderately or extremely while on the drug. Depression continued to affect family life for 79 percent, and it impaired work performance for 72 percent (Reuters, November 30, 1999). Speaking of alternatives to medications, a recent study of 156 people diagnosed with Major Depressive Disorder compared the effects of the antidepressant Zoloft (sertraline), which is similar to Prozac, with sixteen weeks of supervised aerobic exercise sessions. The effects of the medication and exercise were comparable after four months, and after ten months subjects in the exercise group had significantly lower relapse rates than those in the medication group. M. Babyak, et al., Exercise treatment for major depression: Maintenance of therapeutic benefit at 10 months, *Psychosomatic Medicine* 62 (2000): 633–38.

31. Jacobs and Azmitia, Structure and function of the brain serotonin system; B. L. Jacobs and C. A. Fornal, Activity of serotonergic neurons in behaving animals, *Neuropsychopharmacology* 99 (1999): 9–15S.

32. See, for example, F. Chaouloff, Effects of acute physical exercise on central serotonergic systems, *Medicine and Science in Sports and Exercise*

29 (1997): 58–62; L. L. Steinberg, et al., Serum level of serotonin during rest and during exercise in paraplegic patients, *Spinal Cord* 36 (1998): 18–20.

33. R. A. Depue and M. R. Spoont, Conceptualizing a serotonin trait: A behavioral dimension of restraint, *Annals of the New York Academy of Sciences* 487 (1986): 47–62; Jacobs and Azmitia, Structure and function of the brain serotonin system.

34. See, for example, G. F. Weiss, P. Papadakos, K. Knudson, and S. F. Leibowitz, Medial hypothalamic serotonin: Effects on deprivation and norepinephrine-induced eating, *Pharmacology, Biochemistry, and Behavior* 25 (1986): 1223–30.

35. Unlike the serotonergic system, which is unresponsive to stressful conditions, the brain noradrenergic system is responsive to physically arousing stimuli and to tonic stimuli that represent danger. Moreover, there is some evidence that the serotonergic and noradrenergic systems may have an oppositional relationship (Jacobs and Azmitia, Structure and function of the brain serotonin system), and this could be a basis for the reciprocal relationship between energetic and tense arousal at high level of activation, a relationship described previously.

36. R. N. Golden and D. S. Janowsky, Biological theories of depression, in *Depressive disorders: Facts, theories, and treatment models*, ed. B. B. Wolman and G. Stricker (New York: Wiley, 1990); E. T. McNeal and P. Cimbolic, Antidepressants and biochemical theories of depression, *Psychological Bulletin* 99 (1986): 361–74.

37. M. Le Moal and H. Simon, Mesocorticolimbic dopaminergic network: Functional and regulatory roles, *Physiological Reviews* 71 (1992): 155–234.

38. R. A. Depue, M. Luciana, P. Argisi, P. Collins, and A. Leon, Dopamine and structure of personality: Relation of agonist-induced dopamine activity to positive emotionality, *Journal of Personality and Social Psychology* 67 (1994): 485–98.

39. An interesting theory was proposed by D. Tucker and P. Williamson, in which dopamine projections result in a kind of tonic activation similar to tense arousal and interact with norepinephrine projections that produce phasic arousal (like energetic arousal). If this theory is correct, the interaction of these two neurochemical systems could be a basis for the reciprocal interaction of energy and tension described previously (D. M. Tucker and P. A. Williamson, Asymmetric neural

control systems in human self-regulation, *Psychological Review* 91 [1984]: 185–215. See also D. Derryberry and D. M. Tucker, The adaptive basis of the neural hierarchy: Elementary motivational controls on network function, in *Nebraska Symposium on motivation*, ed. R. A. Dienstbier [Lincoln: University of Nebraska Press, 1990]).

40. For example, J. Panksepp offered a plausible hypothesis: "A unitary functional principle underlying opioid function in the brain is the homeostatic reestablishment of baseline conditions in many types of neuronal circuits following stressful perturbations" (J. Panksepp, The neurochemistry of behavior, *Annual Review of Psychology* 37 [1986]: 77–107).

41. D. Hatfield, The mechanisms of exercise-induced psychological states, in *Psychology of sports, exercise and fitness,* ed. L. Diamond (New York: Hemisphere Books, 1991), and M. N. Janal, E. W. D. Colt, W. C. Clark, and M. Glusman, Pain sensitivity, mood and plasma endocrine levels in man following long-distance running: Effects of Naloxone, *Pain* 19 (1984): 13–25.

42. L. W. Role and J. P. Kelly, The brain stem: Cranial nerve nuclei and the monoaminergic systems, in *Principles of neural science,* 3rd ed., ed. E. R. Kandel, J. H. Schwartz, and T. M. Jessell (Norwalk, Conn.: Appleton & Lange, 1991), 681–710.

43. In any analysis of overeating, one must consider evidence about limbic system elements, including the lateral hypothalamus, the so-called feeding center, and the ventromedial hypothalamus, which is associated with satiety. Early dual center theories of feeding control identified these areas of the brain as controlling the motivation to eat and to stop eating. Later research has focused on these structures and others as parts of integrated systems, including various neurochemicals such as norepinephrine, dopamine, serotonin, neuropeptide Y, galanin, and others (J. R. Vasselli and C. A. Maggio, Mechanisms of appetite and body weight regulation, in *Overweight and weight management*, ed. S. Dalton [Gaithersburg, Md.: Aspen Publishers, 1997]).

44. See J. LeDoux, *The emotional brain* (New York: Simon & Schuster, 1996). Even before *The emotional brain* was published, LeDoux's ideas became well known to the general public through Daniel Goleman's highly regarded best-seller, *Emotional intelligence* (New York: Bantam Books, 1995).

45. If that is the case, there is ample evidence of excitatory and inhibitory

influences between the two brain structures to account for the positive and negative relationships between energy and tension (Derryberry and Tucker, Adaptive basis of the neural hierarchy).

46. For example, see R. G. Robinson, Investigating mood disorders following brain injury: An integrative approach using clinical and laboratory studies, *Integrative Psychiatry* 1 (1983): 35–39.

47. See a recent review in A. J. Tomarken and A. D. Keener, Frontal brain asymmetry and depression: A self-regulatory perspective, *Cognition and Emotion* 12 (1998): 387–420.

48. See N. A. Fox, If it's not left, it's right: Electroencephalography asymmetry and the development of emotion, *American Psychologist* 46 (1991): 863–72, and Tomarken and Keener, Frontal brain asymmetry.

49. Another adherent to this idea is David Watson, who coined the well-known terms *positive* and *negative affect*. In *Mood and temperament* (New York: Guilford, 2000) he expanded what previously had been a psychological theory to suggest the importance of this kind of brain asymmetry underlying the two kinds of affect.

Chapter 9   Managing Your Mood

1. R. D. Mattes and M. I. Friedman, Hunger, *Digestive Diseases* 11 (1993): 65–77.

2. J. Mayer, L. F. Monello, and C. C. Seltzer, Hunger and satiety sensation in man, *Postgraduate Medicine* 6 (1965): 97–102.

3. This kind of awareness is especially important, as evidenced by a recent survey carried out by the American Institute for Cancer Research of 1,000 people eighteen years and older. It showed that 34 percent eat what they are used to eating, regardless of changing caloric needs. Also, 26 percent eat everything on their plate, no matter how much is served. This is especially likely to result in weight gain, since there is evidence that portion sizes in restaurants have been getting bigger in recent years, and people are increasingly eating out (Reuters, March 30, 2000).

4. R. E. Thayer, *The origin of everyday moods* (New York: Oxford University Press, 1996).

5. H. Benson, *The relaxation response* (New York: Morrow, 1975).

6. A. Weil, *Breathing: The master key to self-healing*, audio book (Boulder, Colo.: Sounds True, Inc., 1999).

7. For the stimulating breath, Weil instructs: "Breathe in and out rapidly, through your nose, keeping your mouth lightly closed. Inhalation and exhalation should be of equal length, and as short as possible. Get in as many as three cycles per second, if you can do that comfortably. This produces a rapid movement of the diaphragm, which stimulates the movement of a bellows. It is a fairly noisy breath to make." Weil advises that at first you should not do this any longer than fifteen seconds, and after that you should breathe normally. He suggests increasing the time by about five seconds each time you do it, until you have worked up to a full minute.

   For the relaxing breath, Weil instructs: "Inhale through your nose quietly and exhale through your mouth noisily, exhaling around your tongue (it helps to purse your lips). The sound you make when you exhale is a kind of whoosh. Try that a few times so that you get comfortable with exhaling through your mouth and around your tongue.

   Begin the Relaxing Breath by exhaling through your nose completely. Then inhale through your nose to a count of four; hold your breath for a count of seven; and exhale through your mouth for a count of eight. Repeat that for a total of four breath cycles (you will find that this takes little time). What is important here is the ratio of four, seven, and eight for inhalation, hold, and exhalation, respectively. The amount of time you spend doing the four breath cycles is not as important as that ratio. Your exhalation must last for a count of eight, so resist the temptation to blow it all in the first two seconds. Let out a slow, measured breath; then repeat the cycle again. At the end of four breath cycles, just breathe normally without trying to influence the breath" (A. Weil, *A Study guide to breathing: The master key to self-healing* [Boulder, Colo.: Sounds True, Inc.]).

8. T George Harris, The grand-time striders, *Saturday Evening Post*, March/April, 1992.

9. In L. Mundy, contrib. ed. T George Harris, *The complete guide to prayer-walking: A simple path to body-and-soul fitness* (St. Meinrad, Ind.: Abbey Press, 1994).

10. M. Muraven, R. Baumeister, and D. Tice provide experimental evidence that persons who practice self-control become better at future

self-regulation—something like strengthening a muscle (M. Muraven, R. F. Baumeister, and D. M. Tice, Longitudinal improvement of self-regulation through practice: Building self-control strength through repeated exercise, *Journal of Social Psychology* 139 [1999]: 446–57).

References

Abramson, E. 1993. *Emotional eating*. New York: Lexington Books.

Allison, D. B., and S. Heshka. 1993. Emotion and eating in obesity? A critical analysis. *International Journal of Eating Disorders* 13: 289–95.

American Psychiatric Association. 1994. *Diagnostic and statistical manual of mental disorders*. 4th ed. Washington, D.C.

Andres, R. 1995. Body weight and age. In *Eating disorders and obesity: A comprehensive handbook*, ed. K. D. Brownell and C. G. Fairburn, 65–70. New York: Guilford.

Antonuccio, D. O., W. G. Danton, and G. Y. DeNelsky. 1995. Psychotherapy versus medication for depression: Challenging the conventional wisdom with data. *Professional Psychology: Research and Practice* 26: 574–85.

Arnot, Robert. 1997. *Dr. Bob Arnot's revolutionary weight control program*. Boston: Little, Brown.

Arnow, B., J. Kenardy, and W. S. Agras. 1995. The emotional eating scale: The development of a measure to assess coping with negative affect by eating. *International Journal of Eating Disorders* 18: 79–90.

Aronoff, N. J. 1997. Obesity-related eating patterns: Binge-eating disorder and the night-eating syndrome. In *Overweight and weight management*, ed. S. Dalton. Gaithersburg, Md.: Aspen Publishers.

Babyak, M., et al. 2000. Exercise treatment for major depression: Maintenance of therapeutic benefit at 10 months. *Psychosomatic Medicine* 62:633–38.

Bandura, A. 1977. Self-efficacy: Toward a unifying theory of behavior change. *Psychological Review* 84: 191–215.

Barefoot, J. C., B. L. Heitmann, M. J. Helms, R. B. Williams, R. S. Surwit, and I. C. Siegler. 1998. Symptoms of depression and changes in body weight from adolescence to mid-life. *International Journal of Obesity and Related Metabolic Disorders* 22: 688–94.

Bassin, R. B. 1989. The relationship of exercise, self-reported depression and activation level. Master's thesis. California State University, Long Beach.

Baumeister, R. F., T. F. Heatherton, and D. M. Tice. 1994. *Losing control: How and why people fail at self-regulation.* San Diego, Calif.: Academic Press.

Beck, A. T. 1976. *Cognitive therapy and the emotional disorders.* New York: International Universities Press.

Benson, H. 1975. *The relaxation response.* New York: William Morrow.

Benton, D., and D. Owens. 1993. Is raised blood glucose associated with the relief of tension? *Journal of Psychosomatic Research* 37: 723–35.

Beumont, P. J., B. Arthur, J. D. Russell, and S. W. Touyz. 1994. Excessive physical activity in eating disorder patients: Proposals for a supervised exercise program. *International Journal of Eating Disorders* 15: 21–36.

Blaney, P. H. 1986. Affect and memory: A review. *Psychological Bulletin* 99: 229–46.

Blundell, J. E., and N. A. King. 1998. Effects of exercise on appetite control: Loose coupling between energy expenditure and energy intake. *International Journal of Obesity* 22: S22–29.

Brauer, L. H., C. E. Johanson, C. R. Schuster, R. B. Rothman, and H. de Wit. 1996. Evaluation of phentermine and fenfluramine, alone and in combination, in normal, healthy volunteers. *Neuropsychopharmacology* 14: 233–41.

Braun, S. 2000. *The science of happiness.* New York: Wiley.

Bray, G. A., and B. M. Popkin. 1998. Dietary fat does affect obesity! *American Journal of Clinical Nutrition* 68: 1157–73.

Bray, G. A., B. York, and J. DeLany. 1992. A survey of the opinions of obesity experts on the causes and treatment of obesity. *American Journal of Clinical Nutrition* 55: 151–54S.

Brown, G. 2000. *The energy of life.* New York: Free Press.

Brown, W. A. 1984. Use of dexamethasone suppression test in test of depression. In *Neurobiology of mood disorders,* ed. R. M. Post and J. C. Ballenger. Baltimore: Williams and Wilkens.

Bruch, H. 1973. *Eating disorders: Obesity, anorexia nervosa, and the person within*. New York: Basic Books.

Buchwald, D., J. L. Sullivan, and A. L. Komaroff. 1987. Frequency of 'chronic active Epstein-Barr virus infection' in general medical practice. *Journal of the American Medical Association* 257: 2303–7.

Cannon, W. B. 1929/1963. *Bodily changes in pain, hunger, fear and rage*. New York: Harper & Row.

Carver, C. S., S. K. Sutton, and M. F. Scheier. 2000. Action, emotion and personality: Emerging conceptual integration. *Personality and Social Psychology Bulletin* 26: 741–51.

Castonguay, T. W. 1991. Glucocorticoids as modulators in the control of feeding. *Brain Research Bulletin* 27: 423–28.

Cathcart, S., and D. Pritchard. 1998. Relationship between arousal-related moods and episodic tension-type headache: A biopsychological study. *Headache 38*: 214–21.

Chaouloff, F. 1997. Effects of acute physical exercise on central serotonergic systems. *Medicine and Science in Sports and Exercise* 29: 58–62.

Christensen, L. 1993. Effects of eating behavior on mood: A review of the literature. *International Journal of Eating Disorders* 14:171–83.

Christensen, L. 1996. *Diet-behavior relationships*, app. A. Washington, D.C.: American Psychological Association.

Christensen, L., and K. Duncan. 1995. Distinguishing depressed from nondepressed individuals using energy and psychosocial variables. *Journal of Consulting and Clinical Psychology* 63: 495–98.

Clark, L. A., and D. Watson. 1991. Tripartite model of anxiety and depression: Psychometric evidence and taxonomic implications. *Journal of Abnormal Psychology* 100: 316–36.

Cohen, S., D. A. J. Tyrrell, and A. P. Smith. 1991. Psychological stress and susceptibility to the common cold. *New England Journal of Medicine* 325: 606–12.

Cordain, L., R. W. Gotshall, and S. B. Eaton. 1997. Evolutionary aspects of exercise. *World Review of Nutrition Dietetics* 81: 49–60.

Costa, P. T. and R. R. McCrae. 1980. Influence of extraversion and neuroticism on subjective well-being: Happy and unhappy people. *Journal of Personality and Social Psychology* 38: 668–78.

Cousins, S. O. 1998. *Exercise, aging, and health*. New York: Taylor and Francis.

Crews, D. J., and D. M. Landers. 1987. A meta-analytic review of aerobic fitness and reactivity to psychosocial stressors. *Medicine and Science in Sports and Exercise* 19: S114–20.

Czeisler, C. A., et al. 1999. Stability, precision, and near-24–hour period of the human circadian pacemaker. *Science* 284: 2177–81.

Dalton, S., ed. 1997. *Overweight and weight management*. Gaithersburg, Md.: Aspen Publishers.

Dement, W. C. 1999. *The promise of sleep*. New York: Delacorte Press.

DeNeve, K. M., and H. Cooper. 1998. The happy personality: A meta-analysis of 137 traits and subjective well-being. *Psychological Bulletin* 124: 197–229.

Depue, R. A., M. Luciana, P. Argisi, P. Collins, and A. Leon. 1994. Dopamine and structure of personality: Relation of agonist-induced dopamine activity to positive emotionality. *Journal of Personality and Social Psychology* 67: 485–98.

Depue, R. A., and M. R. Spoont. 1986. Conceptualizing a serotonin trait: A behavioral dimension of restraint. *Annals of the New York Academy of Sciences* 487: 47–62.

Derryberry, D., and D. M. Tucker. 1990. The adaptive basis of the neural hierarchy: Elementary motivational controls on network function. In *Nebraska Symposium on Motivation*, ed. R. A. Dienstbier. Lincoln: University of Nebraska Press.

Diener, E., H. Smith, and F. Fujita. 1995. The personality structure of affect. *Journal of Personality and Social Psychology* 69: 130–41.

Dienstbier, R. A. 1991. Behavioral correlates of sympathoadrenal reactivity: The toughness model. *Medicine and Science in Sports and Exercise* 23: 846–52.

———. 1989. Arousal and physiological toughness: Implications for mental and physical health. *Psychological Review* 96: 84–100.

Dillon, K. M. 1992. Popping sealed-air capsules to reduce stress. *Psychological Reports* 71: 243–46.

Dingus, D. F., S. D. Douglas, S. Hamarman, L. Zaugg, and S. Kapoor. 1995. Sleep deprivation and human immune function. *Advances in Neuroimmunology* 5: 97–110.

Dingus, D. F., et al. 1997. Cumulative sleepiness, mood disturbance, and psychomotor vigilance performance decrements during a week of sleep restricted to 4–5 hours per night. *Sleep* 20: 267–77.

Dixon, J. K., J. P. Dixon, and M. Hickey. 1993. Energy as a central factor in the self-assessment of health. *Advances in Nursing Science* 15: 1–12.

Docuyanan, F. M., and R. E. Thayer. 1993. Effectiveness of study time as a function of transitory moods. Paper presented at the annual convention of the American Psychological Association, Toronto, Canada.

Edell, D., with D. Schrieberg. 1999. *Eat, drink, and be merry*. New York: HarperCollins.

Ekkekakis, P., E. E. Hall, and S. J. Petruzzello. 1999. Measuring state anxiety in the context of acute exercise using the State Anxiety Inventory: An attempt to resolve the brouhaha. *Journal of Sport and Exercise Psychology* 21: 205–29.

Ekkekakis, P., E. E. Hall, L. M. Van Landuyt, and S. J. Petruzzello. 2000. Walking in (affective) circles: Can short walks enhance affect? *Journal of Behavioral Medicine* 23: 245–75.

Ekkekakis, P., and S. J. Petruzzello. 1999. Acute aerobic exercise and affect: Current status, problems, and prospects regarding dose-response. *Sports Medicine* 28: 337–74.

Eysenck, H. J. and M. W. Eysenck. 1985. *Personality and individual differences: A natural science approach*. New York: Plenum.

Faith, M. S., D. B. Allison, and A. Geliebter. 1997. Emotional eating and obesity: Theoretical considerations and practical recommendations. In *Overweight and weight management*, ed. S. Dalton. Gaithersburg, Md.: Aspen Publishers.

Farley, F. 1986. The big T in personality. *Psychology Today* 20: 44–52.

Field, T. M. 1998. Massage therapy effects. *American Psychologist* 53: 1270–81.

Flegal, K. M., M. D. Carroll, R. J. Kuczmarski, and C. L. Johnson. 1998. Overweight and obesity in the United States: Prevalence and trends, 1960–1994. *International Journal of Obesity Research Relating to Metabolic Disorders* 22: 39–47.

Ford, E. S., I. B. Ahluwalia, and D. A. Galuski. 2000. Social relationships and cardiovascular disease risk factors: Findings from the third national health and nutrition examination survey. *Preventive Medicine* 30: 83–92.

Fox, N. A. 1991. If it's not left, it's right: Electroencephalography asymmetry and the development of emotion. *American Psychologist* 46: 863–72.

Friedman, M. A., and K. D. Brownell. 1995. Psychological correlates of obesity: Moving to the next research generation. *Psychological Bulletin* 117: 3–20.

Friedman, M., and R. H. Rosenman. 1974. *Type A behavior and your heart.* New York: Knopf.

Ganley, R. M. 1989. Emotion and eating in obesity: A review of the literature. *International Journal of Eating Disorders* 8: 342–61.

Garvey, M. J., and C. B. Schaffer. 1994. Are some symptoms of depression age-dependent? *Journal of Affective Disorders* 32: 247–51.

Gauvin, L., W. J. Rejeski, and J. L. Norris. 1996. A naturalistic study of the impact of acute physical activity on feeling states and affect in women. *Health Psychology* 15: 391–97.

Gauvin, L., W. J. Rejeski, and B. A. Reboussin. 2000. Contributions of acute bouts of vigorous physical activity to explaining diurnal variations in feeling states in active, middle-aged women. *Health Psychology* 19: 365–75.

Gauvin, L., and J. C. Spence. 1996. Physical activity and psychological well-being: Knowledge base, current issues, and caveats. *Nutrition Reviews* 54: S53–65.

Gaylin, W. 1979. *Feelings: Our vital signs.* New York: Ballantine.

Gleim, G.W. 1993. Exercise is not an effective weight loss modality in women. *Journal of the American College of Nutrition* 12: 363–67.

Glick, J. 1999. *Faster: The acceleration of just about everything.* New York: Pantheon Books.

Gold, A. E., K. M. Macleod, I. J. Deary, and B. M. Frier. 1995. Changes in mood during acute hypoglycemia in healthy subjects. *Journal of Personality and Social Psychology* 68: 498–504.

Golden, R. N. and D. S. Janowsky. 1990. Biological theories of depression. In *Depressive disorders: Facts, theories, and treatment models,* ed. B. B. Wolman and G. Stricker. New York: Wiley.

Goleman, D. 1995. *Emotional intelligence.* New York: Bantam Books.

Green, D. P., S. L. Goldman, and P. Salovey. 1993. Measurement error masks bipolarity in affect ratings. *Journal of Personality and Social Psychology* 64: 1029–41.

Green, D. P., and P. Salovey. 1999. In what sense are positive and negative affect independent? A reply to Tellegen, Watson, and Clark. *Psychological Science* 10: 304–6.

Greeno, G. G., and R. R. Wing. 1994. Stress-induced eating. *Psychological Bulletin* 115: 444–64.

Grilo, C. M., S. Shiffman, and R. R. Wing. 1989. Relapse crises and coping among dieters. *Journal of Consulting and Clinical Psychology* 57: 488–95.

Gross, J. J. 1999. Emotion regulation: Past, present, future. *Cognition and Emotion* 13: 551–73.

Haas, Robert. 1994. *Eat smart, think smart.* New York: HarperCollins.

Hager, J. L. 1976. The human respiratory response in state anxiety. Ph.D. diss., Cornell University. *Dissertation Abstracts International* 37: 5423B.

Hall, S. M., R. McGee, C. Tunstall, J. Duffy, and N. Benowitz. 1989. Changes in food intake and activity after quitting smoking. *Journal of Consulting and Clinical Psychology* 57: 81–86.

Harris, T George. 1992. The grand-time striders. *Saturday Evening Post,* March/April.

Hatfield, D. 1991. The mechanisms of exercise-induced psychological states. In *Psychology of Sports, Exercise and Fitness,* ed. L. Diamond. New York: Hemisphere Books.

Heatherton, T. F., C. P. Herman, J. Polivy, G. A. King, and S. T. McGree. 1988. The (mis)measurement of restraint: An analysis of conceptual and psychometric issues. *Journal of Abnormal Psychology* 97: 19–28.

Hepburn, D. A., I. J. Deary, M. Munoz, and B. M. Frier. 1995. Physiological manipulations of psychometric mood factors using acute insulin-induced hypoglycemia in humans. *Personality and Individual Differences* 18: 385–91.

Herman, C. P., and D. Mack. 1975. Restrained and unrestrained eating. *Journal of Personality* 43: 647–60.

Herzog, D. B., K. M. Nussbaum, and A. K. Marmor. 1996. Comorbidity and outcome in eating disorders. *The Psychiatric Clinics of North America* 19: 843–59.

Hicks, R. A., J. Green, and J. Haleblian. 1989. The Thayer Scale response patterns of Type A and Type B college students. *Psychological Reports* 65: 1167–70.

Hill, A. J., and L. Heaton-Brown. 1994. The experience of food craving: A prospective investigation in healthy women. *Journal of Psychosomatic Research* 38: 801–14.

Hirschfeld, R. M., et al. 1997. The National Depressive and Manic-Depressive Association consensus statement on the undertreatment of depression. *Journal of the American Medical Association* 277: 333–40.

Hobson, J. A. 1994. *The chemistry of conscious states.* Boston: Little, Brown.

Hoffman, R. L. 1997. *Intelligent medicine.* New York: Simon & Schuster.

Hsiao, E. T., and R. E. Thayer. 1998. Exercising for mood regulation: The importance of experience. *Personality and Individual Differences* 24: 829–36.

Hubert, H. B., M. Feinleib, P. M. McNamara, and W. P. Castelli. 1983. Obesity as an independent risk factor for cardiovascular disease: A 26–year follow-up of participants in the Framingham Heart Study. *Circulation* 67: 968–77.

Irwin, M., et al. 1996. Partial night sleep deprivation reduces natural killer and cellular immune responses in humans. *Journal of the Federation of the American Societies for Experimental Biology* 10: 643–53

Jackson, I. M. 1998. The thyroid axis and depression. *Thyroid* 8: 951–56.

Jacobs, B. L. 1994. Serotonin, motor activity and depression-related disorders. *American Scientist* 82: 456–63.

Jacobs, B. L., and E. C. Azmitia. 1992. Structure and function of the brain serotonin system. *Physiological Reviews* 72: 165–229.

Jacobs, B. L., and C. A. Fornal. 1999. Activity of serotonergic neurons in behaving animals. *Neuropsychopharmacology* 99: 9–15S

Jacobson, E. 1964. *Anxiety and tension control.* Philadelphia: Lippincott.

Jakicic, J. M., R. R. Wing, B. A. Butler, and R. J. Robertson. 1995. Prescribing exercise in multiple short bouts versus one continuous bout: Effects on adherence, cardiovascular fitness, and weight loss in overweight women. *International Journal of Obesity* 19: 893–901.

Janal, M. N., E. W. D. Colt, W. C. Clark, and M. Glusman. 1984. Pain sensitivity, mood and plasma endocrine levels in man following long-distance running: Effects of Naloxone. *Pain* 19: 13–25.

Jeffery, R. W., and S. A. French. 1998. Epidemic obesity in the United States: Are fast foods and television viewing contributing? *American Journal of Public Health* 88: 277–80.

Johnson, C., and R. Larson. 1982. Bulimia: An analysis of moods and behavior. *Psychosomatic Medicine* 44: 341–51.

Julien, R. M. 1992. *A primer of drug action.* New York: Freeman.

Kandel, E. R. 1991. Disorders of mood: Depression, mania, and anxiety disorders. In *Principles of neural science*, ed. Kandel, et al., 869–86. Norwalk, Conn.: Appleton and Lange.

Kelleher, K. J., T. K. McInerny, W. P. Gardner, G. E. Childs, and R. C.

Wasserman. 2000. Increasing identification of psychosocial problems: 1979–1996. *Pediatrics* 105: 1313–21.

Kenardy, J., B. Arnow, and W. S. Agras. 1996. The aversiveness of specific emotional states associated with binge-eating in obese subjects. *Australian and New Zealand Journal of Psychiatry* 30: 839–44.

Kessler, R. C., et al. 1994. Lifetime and 12–month prevalence of DSM-III-R psychiatric disorders in the United States. *Archives of General Psychiatry* 51: 8–19.

Ketai, R. 1975. Affect, mood, emotion and feeling: Semantic considerations. *American Journal of Psychiatry* 132: 1215–17.

Keys, A., J. Brozek, A. Henschel, O. Mickelsen, and H. L. Taylor. 1950. *The biology of human starvation.* Minneapolis: University of Minnesota Press.

King, N. A., V. J. Burley, and J. E. Blundell. 1994. Exercise-induced suppression of appetite: Effects on food intake and implications for energy balance. *European Journal of Clinical Nutrition* 48: 715–724.

King, N. A., A. Tremblay, and J. E. Blundell. 1996. Effects of exercise on appetite control: Implications for energy balance. *Medicine and Science in Sports and Exercise* 29: 1076–89.

Kirsch, I., and G. Sapirstein. 1998. Listening to Prozac but hearing placebo: A meta-analysis of antidepressant medication. *Prevention and Treatment* 1.

Kleitman, N. 1963. *Sleep and wakefulness,* rev. ed. Chicago: University of Chicago Press.

Laessle, R. G., R. J. Tuschl, B. C. Kotthaus, and K. M. Pirke. 1989. A comparison of the validity of three scales for the assessment of dietary restraint. *Journal of Abnormal Psychology* 98: 504–7.

LaPorte, D. J. 1990. A fatiguing effect in obese patients during partial fasting: Increase in vulnerability to emotion-related events and anxiety. *International Journal of Eating Disorders* 9: 345–55.

Larsen, R. J. 2000. Toward a science of mood regulation. *Psychological Inquiry* 11: 129–41.

Larsen, R. J., and E. Diener. 1992. Promises and problems with the circumplex model of emotion. In *Review of personality and social psychology: Emotion,* vol. 13, ed. M. S. Clark, 25–59. Newbury Park, Calif.: Sage.

Lauderdale, D. S., et al. 1997. Familial determinants of moderate and intense physical activity: A twin study. *Medicine and Science in Sports and Exercise* 29: 1062–68.

Lazarus, R. J. 1991. *Emotion and adaptation*. New York: Oxford University Press.

LeDoux, J. 1996. *The emotional brain*. New York: Simon & Schuster.

Lee, C. D., S. N. Blair, and A. S. Jackson. 1999. Cardiorespiratory fitness, body composition, and all-cause and cardiovascular disease mortality in men. *American Journal of Clinical Nutrition* 69: 373–80.

Le Moal, M., and H. Simon. 1992. Mesocorticolimbic dopaminergic network: Functional and regulatory roles. *Physiological Reviews* 71: 155–234.

Leonard, B. E. 1996. Serotonin receptors and their function in sleep, anxiety disorders and depression. *Psychotherapy and Psychosomatics* 65: 66–75.

Levine, J., P. Baukol, and I. Pavlidis. 1999. The energy expended in chewing gum. *New England Journal of Medicine* 341: 2100.

Levine, J. A., N. L. Eberhardt, and M. D. Jensen. 1999. Role of nonexercise activity thermogenesis in resistance to fat gain in humans. *Science* 283: 212–14.

Lluch, A., P. Hubert, N. A. King, and J. E. Blundell. 2000. Selective effects of acute exercise and breakfast interventions on mood and motivation to eat. *Physiology and Behavior* 68: 515–520.

Long, C. G., J. Smith, M. Midgley, and T. Cassidy. 1993. Over-exercising in anorexic and normal samples: Behaviour and attitudes. *Journal of Mental Health* 2: 321–27.

Ludwig, D. S., et al. 1999. High glycemic index foods, overeating, and obesity. *Pediatrics* 103: E26.

Lykken, D. 1999. *Happiness: What studies of twins show us about nature, nurture and the happiness set-point*. New York: Golden Books.

Maas, J. B. 1998. *Power sleep*. New York: Villard.

McArdle, W. D., F. I. Katch, V. L. Katch. 1991. *Exercise physiology: Energy nutrition and human performance*. Philadelphia: Lea and Febiger.

McAuley, E. 1994. Physical activity and psychsocial outcomes. In *Physical activity, fitness, and health: International proceedings and consensus statement*, ed. C. Bouchard, R. J. Shephard, and T. Stephens. Champaign, Ill.: Human Kenetics Publishers.

McCann, B. S., R. Warnick, and H. Knopp. 1990. Changes in plasma lipids and dietary intake accompanying shifts in perceived workload and stress. *Psychosomatic Medicine* 52: 97–108.

McCrimmon, R. J., B. M. Frier, and I. J. Deary. 1999. Appraisal of mood and personality during hypoglycaemia in human subjects. *Physiology and Behavior* 67: 27–33.

McKenzie, D. C. 1999. Markers of excessive exercise. *Canadian Journal of Applied Physiology* 24: 66–73.

McNair, D. M., M. Lorr, and L. F. Droppleman. 1971. *Manual: Profile of mood states*. San Diego, Calif.: Educational and Industrial Testing Service.

McNeal, E. T., and P. Cimbolic. 1986. Antidepressants and biochemical theories of depression. *Psychological Bulletin* 99: 361–74.

Maddi, S. R. 1999. The personality construct of hardiness: I. Effects on experiencing, coping, and strain. *Consulting Psychology Journal: Practice and Research* 51: 83–94.

Maddi, S. R., D. M. Khoshaba, M. Persico, F. Bleecker, and G. VanArsdall. 1997. Psychosocial correlates of psychopathology in a national sample of the morbidly obese. *Obesity Surgery* 7: 397–404.

Maier, S. F., and L. R. Watkins. 2000. The immune system as a sensory system: Implications for psychology. *Current Directions in Psychological Science* 9: 98–102.

Manson, J. E., et al. 1995. Body weight and mortality among women. *New England Journal of Medicine* 333: 677–85.

Mattes, R. D., and M. I. Friedman. 1993. Hunger. *Digestive Diseases* 11: 65–77.

Matthews, G., D. M. Jones, and A. G. Chamberlain. 1990. Refining the measurement of mood: The UWIST Mood Adjective Checklist. *British Journal of Psychology* 81: 17–42.

Mausner-Dorsch, H., and W. W. Eaton. 200. Psychosocial work environment and depression: Epidemiologic assessment of the demand-control model. *American Journal of Public Health* 90: 1765–70.

Mayer, J., N. B. Marshall, J. J. Vitale, J. H. Christensen, M. B. Mashayekhi, and E. F. Stare. 1954. Exercise, food intake and body weight in normal rats and genetically obese adult mice. *American Journal of Physiology* 177: 544–48.

Mayer, J., L. F. Monello, and C. C. Seltzer. 1965. Hunger and satiety sensation in man. *Postgraduate Medicine* 6: 97–102.

Mayer, J., R. Purnima, and P. M. Kamikhya, 1956. Relation between caloric intake, body weight, and physical work: Studies in an industrial male population in West Bengal. *The American Journal of Clinical Nutrition* 4: 169–75.

Michaud, C. I., J. P. Kahn, N. Musse, C. Burlet, and J. P. Nicolas. 1990. Relationships between critical life events and eating behavior in high-school students. *Stress Medicine* 6: 57–64.

Miller, W. C., and A. K. Lindeman. 1997. The role of diet and exercise in weight management. In *Overweight and weight management,* ed. S. Dalton. Gaithersburg, Md.: Aspen Publishers.

Mitchell, J. E., and M. P. Mussell. 1995. Comorbidity and binge eating disorder. *Addictive Behaviors* 20: 725–32.

Mokdad, A. H., et al. 1999. The spread of the obesity epidemic in the United States, 1991–1998. *Journal of the American Medical Association* 282: 1519–22.

Montplaisir, J., and R. Godbout, eds. 1990. *Sleep and biological rhythms.* New York: Oxford University Press.

Morgan, W. P., 1994. Physical activity, fitness and depression. In *Physical activity, fitness, and health: International proceedings and consensus statement,* ed. C. Bouchard, R. J. Shephard, and T. Stephens, 851–67. Champaign, Ill.: Human Kenetics Publishers.

Morgan, W. P., and M. L. Pollock. 1978. Psychological characterization of the elite distance runner. *Annals of the New York Academy of Science* 301: 382–403.

Mundy, L. (contrib. ed., T George Harris). 1994. *The complete guide to prayer-walking: A simple path to body-and-soul fitness.* St. Meinrad, Ind.: Abbey Press.

Muraven, M., R. F. Baumeister, and D. M. Tice. 1999. Longitudinal improvement of self-regulation through practice: Building self-control strength through repeated exercise. *The Journal of Social Psychology* 139: 446–57.

Murray, E. J. 1965. *Sleep, dreams, and arousal.* New York: Appleton-Century-Crofts.

Must, A., et al. 1999. The disease burden associated with overweight and obesity. *Journal of the American Medical Association* 282: 1523–29.

National Task Force on the Prevention and Treatment of Obesity. 1996. Long-term pharmacotherapy in the management of obesity. *Journal of the American Medical Association* 276: 1907–15.

Nesse, R. M. 1999. The evolution of hope and despair. *Social Research* 66: 429–69.

Nolen-Hoeksema, S. K. 1990. *Women and depression.* Stanford, Calif.: Stanford University Press.

Nowlis, V. 1965. Research with the Mood Adjective Check List. In *Affect, cognition, and personality*, ed. S. S. Tomkins and C.E. Izard, 352–89. New York: Springer.

Nowlis, V,. and H. H. Nowlis. 1956. The description and analysis of moods. *Annals of the New York Academy of Science* 65: 345–55.

O'Connor, P. J., C. X. Bryant, J. P. Veltri, and S. M. Gebhardt. 1993. State anxiety and ambulatory blood pressure following resistance exercise in females. *Medicine and Science in Sports and Exercise* 25: 516–21.

O'Connor, P. J., S. J. Petruzzello, K. A. Kubitz, and T. L. Robinson. 1995. Anxiety responses to maximal exercise testing. *British Journal of Sports Medicine* 29: 97–102.

Osmond, H., R. Mullaly, and C. Bisbee. 1985. Mood pain: A comparative study of clinical pain and depression. *Journal of Orthomolecular Psychiatry* 14: 5–12.

Owens, D. S., P. Y. Parker, and D. Benton. 1997. Blood glucose and subjective energy following cognitive demand. *Physiology and Behavior* 62: 471–78.

Owens, H., and J. S. Maxmen. 1979. Mood and affect: A semantic confusion. *American Journal of Psychiatry* 136: 97–99.

Panksepp, J. 1986. The neurochemistry of behavior. *Annual Review of Psychology* 37: 77–107.

Parkinson, B., and P. Totterdell. 1999. Classifying affect-regulation strategies. *Cognition and Emotion* 13: 277–303.

Peeke, P. 2000. *Fight fat after forty*. New York: Viking.

Pepper, G. M., and D. T. Krieger. 1984. Hypothalamic-pituitary-adrenal abnormalities in depression: Their possible relation to central mechanisms regulating ACTH release. In *Neurobiology of Mood Disorders*, ed. R. M. Post and J. C. Ballenger. Baltimore: Williams and Wilkens.

Pert, C. B. 1997. *Molecules of emotion*. New York: Scribner.

Pervin, L. A., ed. 1989. *Goal concepts in personality and social psychology*. Hilldale, N.J.: Erlbaum.

Petruzzello, S. J., and D. M. Landers. 1994. State anxiety reduction and exercise: Does hemispheric activation reflect such changes? *Medicine Science in Sports and Exercise* 26: 1028–35.

Petruzzello, S. J., D. M. Landers, B. D. Hatfield, K. A. Kubitz, and W. Salazar. 1991. A meta-analysis on the anxiety-reducing effects of acute and chronic exercise. *Sports Medicine* 11: 143–82.

Physical activity and health: A report of the surgeon general. 1996. Atlanta, Ga.:

U.S. Department of Health and Human Services, Centers for Disease Control and Prevention, National Center for Chronic Disease Prevention and Health Prevention, President's Council on Physical Fitness and Sports.

Pilcher, J. J., and A. I. Huffcutt. 1996. Effects of sleep deprivation on performance: A meta-analysis. *Sleep* 19: 318–26.

Popless-Vawter, S., C. Brandau, and J. Straub. 1998. Triggers of overeating and related intervention strategies for women who weight cycle. *Applied Nursing Research* 11: 69–76.

Pronk, N. P., S. F. Crouse, and J. J. Rohack. 1995. Maximal exercise and acute mood response in women. *Physiology and Behavior* 57: 1–4

Pronk, N. P., and R. R. Wing. 1994. Physical activity and long-term maintenance of weight loss. *Obesity Research* 2: 587–99.

Raglin, J. S., P. E. Turner, and F. Eksten. 1993. State anxiety and blood pressure following 30 minutes of leg ergometry or weight training. *Medicine and Science in Sports and Exercise* 9: 1044–48.

Raglin, J. S., and M. Wilson. 1996. State anxiety following 20 minutes of bicycle ergometric exercise at selected intensities. *International Journal of Sports Medicine* 17: 467–71.

Rand, C. S. W., A. M. C. Macgregor, and A. J. Stunkard. 1997. The night-eating syndrome in the general population and among postoperative obesity surgery patients. *International Journal of Eating Disorders* 22: 65–69.

Revelle, W. 1993. Manipulations and measurement of arousal: Within and between—subject evidence for two components of arousal. Paper presented at the meeting of the International Society for the Study of Individual Differences, Baltimore.

Rippe, J. M., and S. Hess. 1998. The role of physical activity in the prevention and management of obesity. *Journal of the American Dietetic Association* 98: S31–38.

Robins, L. N., B. Z. Locke, and D. A. Regier. 1991. An overview of psychiatric disorders in America. In *Psychiatric disorder in America: The epidemiologic catchment area study*, ed. L. N. Robins and D. A. Regier. New York: Free Press.

Robins, L. N., et al. 1984. Lifetime prevalence of specific psychiatric disorders in three sites. *Archives of General Psychiatry* 41: 949–58.

Robinson, J. P., and G. Godbey. 1997. *Time for life: The surprising ways Amer-*

icans use their time. University Park: The Pennsylvania State University Press.

Robinson, M. D. 2000. The reactive and prospective functions of mood: Its role in linking daily experiences and cognitive well-being. *Cognition and Emotion* 14: 145–76.

Robinson, R. G. 1983. Investigating mood disorders following brain injury: An integrative approach using clinical and laboratory studies. *Integrative Psychiatry* 1: 35–39.

Rodin, J. 1992. *Body traps*. New York: Morrow.

Role, L. W., and J. P. Kelly. 1991 The brain stem: Cranial nerve nuclei and the monoaminergic systems. In *Principles of neural science*, 3rd ed., ed. E. R. Kandel, J. H. Schwartz, and T. M. Jessell, 681–710. Norwalk, Conn.: Appleton and Lange.

Rose, G. A., and R. T. Williams. 1961. Metabolic studies of large and small eaters. *British Journal of Nutrition* 15: 1–9.

Rubadeau, J. 1976. The relationship between self-esteem, activation levels, and other situational determinants. Master's thesis. California State University, Long Beach.

Russell, J. A. 1980. A circumplex model of affect. *Journal of Personality and Social Psychology* 39: 1161–78.

Rutledge, T., and W. Linden. 1998. To eat or not to eat: Affective and physiological mechanisms in the stress-eating relationship. *Journal of Behavioral Medicine* 21: 221–40.

Ryan, R. M., C. M. Frederick, D. Lepes, N. Rubio, and K. M. Sheldon. 1997. Intrinsic motivation and exercise adherence. *International Journal of Sports Psychology* 28: 335–54.

Saklofske, D. H., G. C. Blomme, and I. W. Kelly. 1992. The effect of exercise and relaxation on energetic and tense arousal. *Personality and Individual Differences* 13: 623–25.

Samparas, K., et al. 1999. Genetic and environmental influences on total-body and central abdominal fat: The effect of physical activity in female twins. *Annals of Internal Medicine* 130: 873–82.

Scully, D., J. Kremer, M. M. Meade, R. Graham, and K. Dudgeon. 1998. Physical exercise and psychological well-being: A critical review. *British Journal of Sports Medicine* 32: 111–20

Sears, B. 1995. *The zone: A dietary road map*. New York: HarperCollins.

Selye, H. 1956. *The stress of life*. Toronto and London: McGraw-Hill.

Serdula, M. K., et al. 1999. Prevalence of attempting weight loss and strategies for controlling weight. *Journal of the American Medical Association* 282: 1353–58.

Shephard, R. J. 1997. What is the optimal type of physical activity to enhance health? *British Journal of Sports Medicine* 31: 277–84.

Smith, A., M. Thomas, J. Kent, and K. Nicholson. 1998. Effects of the common cold on mood and performance. *Psychoneuroendocrinology* 23: 733–39.

Somer, E. 1995. *Food and mood.* New York: Holt.

Spielberger, C. D. 1983. *Manual for the State-Trait Anxiety Inventory (form Y).* Palo Alto, Calif.: Consulting Psychologists Press.

Stark, P., and C. D. Hardison. 1985. A review of multicenter controlled studies of Fluoxetine vs. Imipramine and placebo in outpatients with Major Depressive Disorder. *Journal of Clinical Psychiatry* 46: 53–58.

Steinberg, L. L., et al. 1998. Serum level of serotonin during rest and during exercise in paraplegic patients. *Spinal Cord* 36: 18–20.

Stephens, T., and C. L. Craig. 1990. *The well-being of Canadians: Highlights of the 1988 Campbell's Survey.* Ottawa: Canadian Fitness and Lifestyle Research Institute.

Steptoe, A., et al. 1998. The effect of life stress on food choice. In *"The nation's diet": The social science of food choice,* ed. A. Murcott. London: Longman.

Steptoe, A., and S. Cox. 1988. Acute effects of aerobic exercise on mood. *Health Psychology* 7: 329–40.

Steptoe, A., J. Kimbell, and P. Basford. 1998. Exercise and the experience and appraisal of daily stressors: A naturalistic study. *Journal of Behavioral Medicine* 21: 363–74.

Steptoe, A., Z. Lipsey, and J. Wardle. 1998. Stress, hassles and variations in alcohol consumption, food choice and physical exercise: A diary study. *British Journal of Health Psychology* 3: 51–63.

Steptoe, A., T. S. Pollard, and J. Wardle. 1995. Development of a measure of the motives underlying the selection of food: The Food Choice Questionnaire. *Appetite* 25: 267–84.

Stevens, J., J. Cai, E. R. Pamuk, D. F. Williamson, M. J. Thun, and J. L. Wood. 1998. The effect of age on the association between body-mass index and mortality. *New England Journal of Medicine* 338: 1–7.

Stokes, P. E. 1993. Fluoxetine: A five-year review. *Clinical Therapeutics* 15: 216–43.

Stone, A. A., J. M. Neale, D. S. Cox, A. Napoli, H. Valdimarsdottir, and E. Kennedy-Moore. 1994. Daily events are associated with secretory immune response to an oral antigen in men. *Health Psychology* 13: 440–46.

Stone, A. A., et al. 1987. Evidence that secretory IgA antibody is associated with daily mood. *Journal of Personality and Social Psychology* 52: 988–93.

Stunkard, A. J., M. H. Fernstrom, R. A. Price, E. Buss, E. Frank, and D. J. Kupfer. 1991. Weight change in depression: Influence of "disinhibition" is mediated by body mass and other variables. *Psychiatry Research* 38: 197–200.

Stunkard, A. J., W. J. Grace, and H. G. Wolff. 1955. The night-eating syndrome: A pattern of food intake among certain obese patients. *American Journal of Medicine* 19: 78–86.

Stunkard, A. J., and S. Messick. 1985. A three-factor eating questionnaire to measure dietary restraint, disinhibition and hunger. *Journal of Psychosomatic Research* 29, 71–83.

Stunkard, A. J., et al. 1996. Binge eating disorder and the night-eating syndrome. *International Journal of Obesity* 20: 1–6.

Suzuki, S. 1970. *Zen mind, beginner's mind.* New York: Weatherhill.

Tate, A. K., and S. J. Petruzzello. 1995. Varying the intensity of acute exercise: Implications for changes in affect. *Journal of Sports Medicine and Physical Fitness* 35: 295–302.

Taubes, G. 1998. As obesity rates rise, experts struggle to explain why. *Science* 280: 1367–68.

Tavris, C. 1989. *Anger: The misunderstood emotion,* rev. ed. New York: Simon & Schuster.

Taylor, S. E., L. C. Klein, B. P. Lewis, T. L. Gruenewald, R. A. R. Gurung, and J. A. Updegraff. 2000. Biobehavioral responses to stress in females: Tend-and-befriend, not fight-or-flight. *Psychological Review* 107: 411–29.

Thayer, R. E. 1970. Activation states as assessed by verbal report and four psychophysiological variables. *Psychophysiology* 7: 86–94.

———. 1978a. Factor analytic and reliability studies on the Activation-Deactivation Adjective Check List. *Psychological Reports* 42: 747–56.

———. 1978b. Toward a psychological theory of multidimensional activation (arousal). *Motivation and Emotion* 2: 1–34.

———. 1987a. Energy, tiredness, and tension effects of a sugar snack versus moderate exercise. *Journal of Personality and Social Psychology* 52: 119–25.

————. 1987b. Problem perception, optimism, and related states as a function of time of day (diurnal rhythm) and moderate exercise: Two arousal systems in interaction. *Motivation and Emotion* 11: 19–36.

————. 1989. *The biopsychology of mood and arousal.* New York: Oxford University Press.

————. 1996. *The origin of everyday moods.* New York: Oxford University Press.

Thayer, R. E., J. R. Newman, and T. M. McClain. 1994. The self-regulation of mood: Strategies for changing a bad mood, raising energy, and reducing tension. *Journal of Personality and Social Psychology* 67: 910–25.

Thayer, R. E., D. P. Peters, P. J. Takahashi, and A. M. Birkhead-Flight. 1993. Mood and behavior (smoking and sugar snacking) following moderate exercise: A partial test of self-regulation theory. *Personality and Individual Differences* 14: 97–104.

Thayer, R. E., P. J. Takahashi, and J. A. Pauli. 1988. Multidimensional arousal states, diurnal rhythms, cognitive and social processes, and extraversion. *Personality and Individual Differences* 9: 15–24.

Tice, D. M., and E. Bratslavsky. 2000. Giving in to feel good: The place of emotion regulation in the context of general self-control. *Psychological Inquiry* 11: 149–59.

Toffler, A. 1970. *Future shock.* New York: Random House.

Tomarken, A. J., and A. D. Keener. 1998. Frontal brain asymmetry and depression: A self-regulatory perspective. *Cognition and Emotion* 12: 387–420.

Tomkins, S. S., and C. E. Izard, eds. 1965. *Affect, cognition, and personality.* New York: Springer.

Toth, M. J., and E. T. Poehlman. 1996. Effects of exercise on daily energy expenditure. *Nutrition Reviews* 54: S140–48.

Tucker, D. M., and P. A. Williamson. 1984. Asymmetric neural control systems in human self-regulation. *Psychological Review* 91: 185–215.

Tuomisto, T., M. T. Tuomisto, M. Hetherington, and R. Lappalainen. 1998. Reasons for initiation and cessation of eating in obese men and women and the affective consequences of eating in everyday situations. *Appetite* 30: 211–22.

Twenge, J. M. 2000. The age of anxiety?: The birth cohort change in anxiety and neuroticism, 1952–1993. *Journal of Personality and Social Psychology* 79: 1007–21.

Valdimarsdottir, H. B. and D. H. Bovbjerg. 1997. Positive and negative mood: Association with natural killer cell activity. *Psychology and Health:* 12, 319–27.

van Eck, M. M., and N. A. Nicolson. 1994. Perceived stress and salivary cortisol in daily life. *Annals of Behavioral Medicine* 16: 221–27.

Van Strien, T. 1995. In defense of psychosomatic theory: A critical analysis of Allison and Heshka's critical analysis. *International Journal of Eating Disorders* 17: 299–304.

Van Strien, T., J. E. R. Frijters, G. P. A. Bergers, and P. B. Defares. 1986. The Dutch Eating Behavior Questionnaire (DEBQ) for assessment of restrained, emotional, and external eating behavior. *International Journal of Eating Disorders* 5: 295–315.

Vasselli, J. R., and C. A. Maggio. 1997. Mechanisms of appetite and body weight regulation. In *Overweight and weight management*, ed. S. Dalton. Gaithersburg, Md.: Aspen Publishers.

Wake up America: A national sleep alert. 1993. Report of the National Commission on Sleep Disorders Research, vol. 1. Washington, D.C.: U. S. Department of Health and Human Services.

Watson, D. 2000. *Mood and temperament.* New York: Guilford.

Watson, D., and A. Tellegen. 1985. Toward a consensual structure of mood. *Psychological Bulletin* 98: 219–35.

Watson, D., D. Wiese, J. Vaidya, and A. Tellegen. 1999. Two general activation systems of affect: Structural findings, evolutionary considerations, and psychobiological evidence. *Journal of Personality and Social Psychology* 76: 820–38.

Watson, D. L., and R. G. Tharp. 1997. *Self-directed behavior.* Pacific Grove, Calif.: Brooks/Cole.

Wegner, D. M., and J. W. Pennebaker, eds. 1993. *Handbook of mental control.* Englewood Cliffs, N.J.: Prentice-Hall.

Wehr, T. A. 1990. Effects of wakefulness and sleep on depression and mania. In *Sleep and biological rhythms*, ed. J. Montplaisir and R. Godbout, 42–86. New York: Oxford University Press.

Weil, A. 1999. *Breathing: The master key to self-healing.* Audio book. Boulder, Colo.: Sounds True, Inc.

Weingarten, H. P., and D. Elston. 1991. Food cravings in a college population. *Appetite* 17: 167–75.

Weiss, G. F., P. Papadakos, K. Knudson, and S. F. Leibowitz. 1986. Medial hypothalamic serotonin: Effects on deprivation and norepinephrine-induced eating. *Pharmacology, Biochemistry, and Behavior* 25: 1223–30.

Weyerer, S., and B. Kupfer. 1994. Physical exercise and psychological health. *Sports Medicine* 17: 108–16.

Wickelgren, I. 1998. Obesity: How big a problem? *Science* 280: 1364–67.

Willett, W. C. 1998a. Dietary fat and obesity: An unconvincing relation. *American Journal of Clinical Nutrition* 68: 1149–50.

————. 1998b. Is dietary fat a major determinant of body fat? *American Journal of Clinical Nutrition* 67: 556–62S.

Wing, R. R., S. Shiffman, R. G. Drapkin, C. M. Grilo, and M. McDermott. 1995. Moderate versus restrictive diets: Implications for relapse. *Behavior therapy* 26: 5–24.

Wright, R. A., and J. W. Brehm. 1989. Energization and goal attractiveness. In *Goal concepts in personality and social psychology*, ed. L. A. Pervin, 169–210. Hillsdale, N.J.: Erlbaum.

Wu, J., et al. 1999. Prediction of antidepressant effects of sleep deprivation by metabolic rates in the ventral anterior cingulate and medial prefrontal cortex. *American Journal of Psychiatry* 156: 1149–58.

Yeung, R. R. 1996. The acute effects of exercise on mood states. *Journal of psychosomatic research* 40: 123–41.

Yik, M. S. M., J. A. Russell, and L. F. Barrett. 1999. Structure of self-reported current affect: Integration and beyond. *Journal of Personality and Social Psychology* 77: 600–619.

Zweifel, J. E., and W. H. O'Brien. 1997. A meta-analysis of the effect of hormone replacement therapy upon depressed mood. *Psychoneuroendocrinology* 22: 189–212.

Index

research *(continued)*
  on mood, 34, 52, 122–24,
    126–28, 181n. 2
  on night-eating syndrome,
    118–19
  on obesity, 16–18
  on overeating, 52, 56–58
  on personality types, 65–67
  on physical illness, 126–27
  popular diets and, 198n. 3 (50),
    199n. 4 (50)
  on self-esteem, 42
  on sleep, 128–29, 191n. 12
    (32), 223n. 30 (128)
  on stress, 24–25, 64, 189n. 51
    (27), 208n. 39 (63), 208n.
    40 (64), 209n. 43 (65)
  on stress management, 43
  on sweets vs. exercise, 79–82
  on triggers to overeating, 56–58
resistance training and mood,
    40–41
respiratory system, 138
rest, food substituted for, 101
restaurants and portion size, 232n.
    3 (164)
resting metabolic rate, 46
restrained eaters. *See* diets
reticular activating system, 149–50
Rippe, James, 46
Robinson, Michael, 217n. 21 (97)
Roper polls, 24
Rubadeau, Joan, 42
runners, 41
Russell, James, 91–92
Rutledge, Thomas, 66, 210n. 46
    (66), 211n. 48 (66)

sadness, 97
Salovey, P., 216n. 11 (92)
satiety, 164, 203n. 19 (55), 230n.
    43 (150)
Sauter, Steve, 22
schedule. *See* energy cycles
Science, 16, 31
science behind popular diets
    books, 50, 198n. 3 (50),
    199n. 4 (50)
Seasonal Affective Disorder
    (SAD), 115, 146
self-affirmations, 174
self-awareness
  of caloric needs, 231n. 3 (164)
  eating slowly, 164
  of energy cycles, 119–21,
    160–61
  of habitual behaviors, 78
  monitoring tension and energy,
    158–70
self-control, 11–12
self-efficacy, 42, 103
self-esteem
  depression and, 105
  energy and, 34, 196n. 38 (42)
  self-awareness of, 164–66
  weight-loss maintenance and,
    47
self-medication. *See* self-regulation
self-observation, 119–21
self-perceptions of overweight,
    183n. 1, 184n. 2
self-regulation. *See also* mood;
    tense tiredness
  alcohol and, 125–26
  common behavior of, 4, 155

ABOUT THE AUTHOR

Robert E. Thayer is the author of *The Biopsychology of Mood and Arousal* and *The Origin of Everyday Moods* (New York: Oxford University Press, 1989, 1996). He is professor of psychology at California State University, Long Beach, where he teaches "The Psychology of Mood," among other courses. His work is widely cited in the scientific literature (for example, he is a Citation Classic author), as well as in the popular science media, where his research has been discussed in hundreds of magazine and newspaper articles. He lives in Seal Beach, California, and his e-mail address is: mood@csulb.edu.